Medical Management of Eating Disorders
A Practical Handbook for Health Care Professionals

This is a practical guide to the medical complications and treatment of anorexia nervosa and related eating disorders. A user-friendly structure allows the reader to access information on the basis of physical complaint (e.g. chest pain) or body system (e.g. neurological or respiratory). Practical guidance is provided on history taking, physical and laboratory examinations, and looking after special categories of patients, such as prepubertal patients, males, adolescents, and pregnant females. The principles and practice of treatment are covered fully, including medical and nutritional therapies. Psychiatric and psychological issues are also addressed, and details of specific psychological therapies are provided. The text is supplemented with diagnostic color photographs of important physical manifestations of eating disorders. Although the text is suitable for all health care professionals looking after these patients, special information is provided for general practitioners, nursing staff, family carers, and the patients themselves.

LAIRD BIRMINGHAM is Professor of Psychiatry at the University of British Columbia, Canada, where he is also an associate member of the Departments of Medicine, Health Care and Epidemiology, and Pharmacology and Clinical Therapeutics. He was Director of the Division of General Internal Medicine at St Paul's Hospital from 1983 until 2000. He is Medical Director of the Eating Disorders Program and leader of the BC Eating Disorder Epidemiology Project in the Center for Health Evaluation and Outcome Sciences as well as British Columbia Provincial Director for Eating Disorders. He has worked in the area of anorexia nervosa and other eating disorders for over 20 years. He has published 70 refereed articles in scientific journals, written seven invited chapters or commissioned articles, and edited four books.

PIERRE BEUMONT has been Professor of Psychiatry at the University of Sydney, Australia, since 1975, and is also Honorary Professor of Psychology. Previously he was Lecturer in Psychiatry at Oxford University, and Senior Lecturer and Acting Head at the University of Cape Town. He was Head of Department in Sydney University from 1975 to 2000. He has worked in the area of anorexia nervosa and other eating disorders for over 30 years. He has published 150 refereed articles in scientific journals, written 96 invited chapters or commissioned articles, and edited four books. More than half have related to anorexia nervosa. In 2001 he was appointed a Member of the Order of Australia in recognition of his work in anorexia nervosa.

Medical Management of Eating Disorders

A Practical Handbook for Health Care Professionals

C. LAIRD BIRMINGHAM
University of British Columbia

PIERRE J. V. BEUMONT
University of Sydney

With invited contributions by
RICHARD CRAWFORD, DEBORAH HODGSON,
MICHAEL KOHN, PETA MARKS, JAMES MITCHELL,
SUE PAXTON, JORGE PINZON, INGRID TYLER,
CHRISTOPHER THORNTON, STEPHEN TOUYZ, AND
ALISON WAKEFIELD

Additional comments by
ELLIOT GOLDNER, WALTER VANDEREYCKEN, AND
DAVID BEN-TOVIM

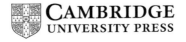

CAMBRIDGE
UNIVERSITY PRESS

PUBLISHED BY THE PRESS SYNDICATE OF THE UNIVERSITY OF CAMBRIDGE
The Pitt Building, Trumpington Street, Cambridge, United Kingdom

CAMBRIDGE UNIVERSITY PRESS
The Edinburgh Building, Cambridge CB2 2RU, UK
40 West 20th Street, New York, NY 10011–4211, USA
477 Williamstown Road, Port Melbourne, VIC 3207, Australia
Ruiz de Alarcón 13, 28014 Madrid, Spain
Dock House, The Waterfront, Cape Town 8001, South Africa

http://www.cambridge.org

First published 2004

Printed in the United Kingdom at the University Press, Cambridge

Typeface Times 10/13 pt.   *System* LATEX 2$_\varepsilon$ [TB]

A catalog record for this book is available from the British Library

Library of Congress Cataloging in Publication data

Medical management of eating disorders: a practical handbook for health care
professionals / by C. Laird Birmingham and Pierre J.V. Beumont; with invited
contributions by Richard Crawford . . . [*et al.*]; forewords by Christopher Fairburn,
Manfred Fichter, and Joel Yager; additional comments by Elliot Goldner . . . [*et al.*].
p.   cm.
Includes bibliographical references and index.
ISBN 0 521 54662 1 paperback
1. Eating disorders. 2. Eating disorders – Complications. I. Beumont, Pierre J. V.
II. Title.
RC552.E18B515   2004
616.85′26–dc22   2003062624

ISBN 0 521 54662 1 paperback

This book is dedicated to the memory of Professor Peter Beumont, who died October 1, 2003. He was a wonderful husband, father, grandfather, psychiatrist, academic, and thinker. He will be greatly missed.

Contents

Color plates

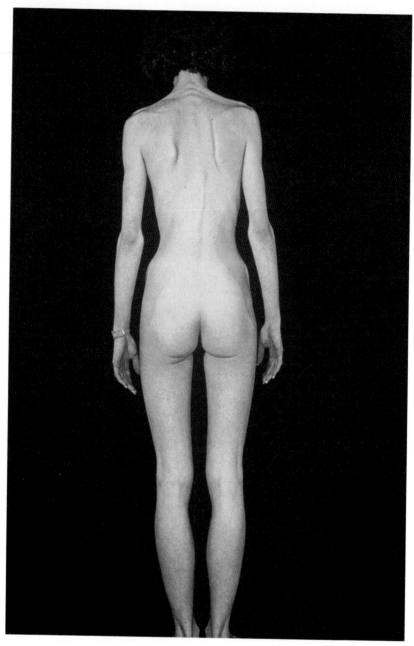

Plates 1a and 1b. Wasting. Note the generalized muscle wasting in addition to the markedly reduced body fat. Muscle wasting is often best assessed by wasting of the temporal muscle, the prominence of the scapulae and the ribs, the obvious lower rib margin, the increased prominence of the anterior superior iliac spine, and wasting of the gluteal muscles.

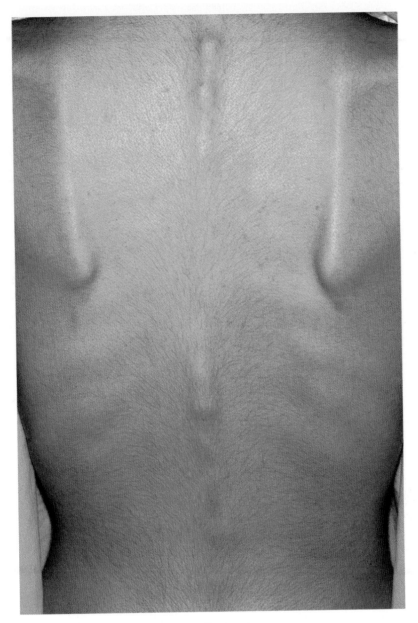

Plate 1b. (cont.)

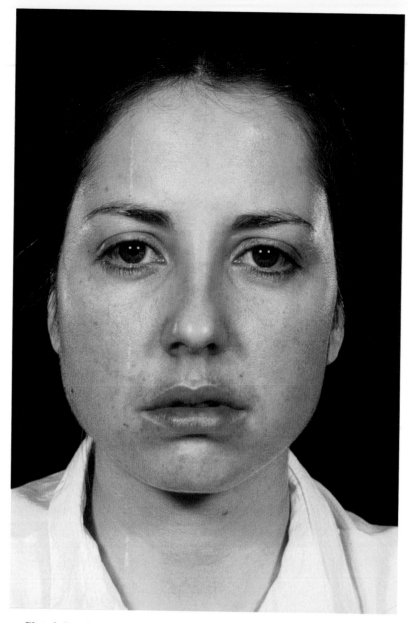

Plate 2. Parotid hypertrophy. The parotid gland is also enlarged in mumps. The parotid gland is about the size of a small oyster. It lies just in front of the ear and above the line of the jaw. When it is enlarged, the face looks wider and the ears stick out a little. Sometimes, but not always, there is a clear line demarcating the edge of the parotid. The parotid can be mildly enlarged with just protein-calorie malnutrition, but it is usually and particularly enlarged with vomiting. If vomiting becomes more frequent, the parotid may rapidly enlarge and become mildly painful and tender to the touch. Stensen's duct, which drains the salivary fluid from the parotid gland into the mouth, is often seen to be more prominent with purging. It is seen inside the mouth just above the second lower molar. It appears as a little prominence with a cavity in its middle. The submandibular glands that lie just below the jaw at a point near the corners of the mouth are enlarged just like the parotid gland.

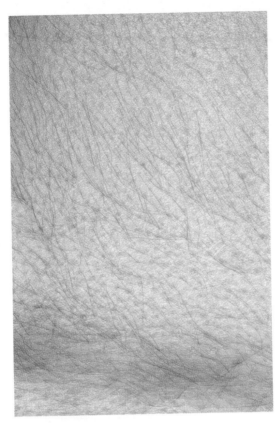

Plate 3. Lanugo hair. This develops at low weight and is similar to the fine hair seen on newborns. It is best appreciated on the abdomen and back. Lanugo hair takes on the same color as the normal hair of the patient. It disappears with recovery.

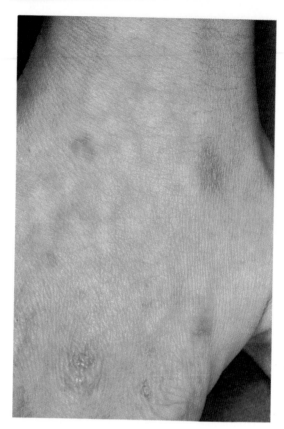

Plate 4. Russell's sign. Named after Professor Gerald Russell, who first described the sign. The scars over the back of the hand result from habitual use of the hand to induce purging. If the hand is not used to induce purging, it will not be present (very often these days patients induce vomiting by will alone). The scars will not disappear.

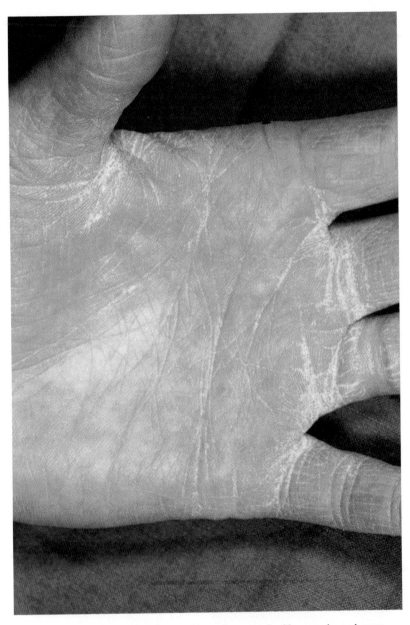

Plate 5. Acrodermatitis. Acrodermatitis can be recognized by very dry and somewhat scaly skin on the palms and soles. Other skin may also be dry and scaly, but usually not to the same degree. A change in taste and an increased difficulty in healing skin abrasions are other clues to an underlying zinc deficiency.

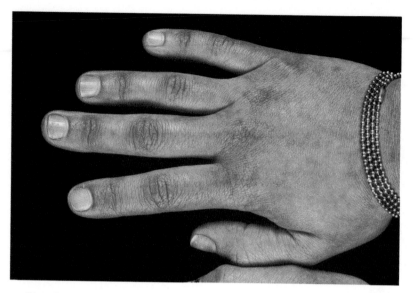

Plate 6. Acrocyanosis. The blue/purple hue of the ends of the extremities is often obvious but overlooked. It is caused by reduced blood flow to the extremities as a result of vasoconstriction due to cold stress and volume depletion. It disappears early in treatment.

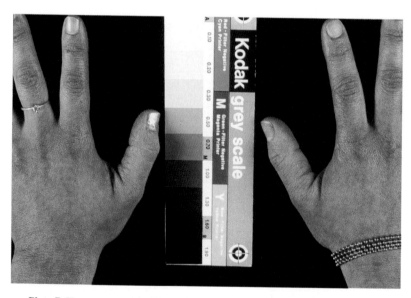

Plate 7. Hypercarotenemia. The patient's body is yellow but, unlike in jaundice, the eyes remain white. Compare your hand with that of the patient, as the light is often dim in examining areas and hospital drapes are often yellow. Carotene bound to elastin in the tissues causes no symptoms, so the patient should not complain of any that relate to hypercarotenemia.

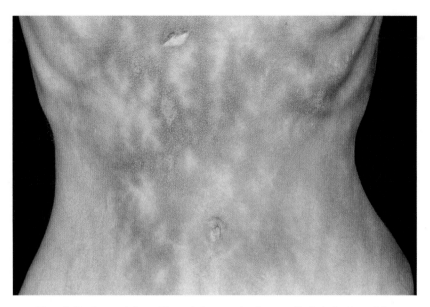

Plate 8. Erythema ab igne. The rash is a poorly circumscribed, darkening of the area of the body to which the patient habitually applies heat. It is without symptoms and does not vary from day to day. It is usually present over the lower back or the abdomen. It is permanent.

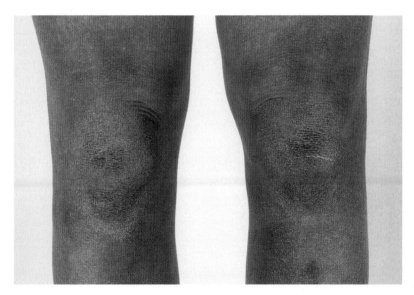

Plate 9. Pellagra. A dark, flaky rash over the front of the lower extremites should raise the suspicion of pellagra.

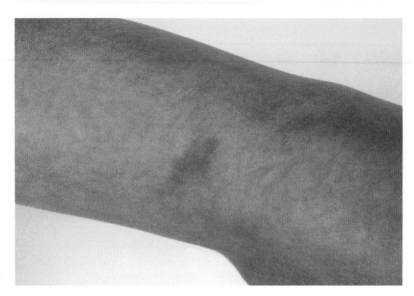

Plate 10. Ecchymoses. Bleeding into the tissues is very common in AN but infrequent in BN. If the bruising is tender, then it is likely to be unrelated to the eating disorder. Hemoglobin is broken down to bilirubin and biliverdin, so the ecchymoses will turn from red to yellow to green in the normal course of things. Scurvy causes easy bleeding and bruising, but it usually presents with small hemorrhages around the hair follicles of the thighs and bleeding from the gums before large ecchymoses occur.

Contributors

Pierre Joseph Victor Beumont, AM, MB, ChB, MSc, MPhil, FRCP(Edin), FRACP, FRC(Psych), FRANZCP, DPM
Professor of Psychiatry and Honorary Professor of Psychology, University of Sydney, Sydney, NSW, Australia
Academic Head, Department of Psychiatry, Royal Prince Alfred Hospital Director, Eating and Dieting Disorders Services, Wesley Hospital and Carlingford Day Centre, Wesley Mission, Sydney, NSW, Australia
Department of Psychological Medicine, University of Sydney, Sydney, NSW, Australia

Carl Laird Birmingham, MD, BSc, MHSc, FRCPC, FACP, ABIM
Professor and Director, Eating Disorders Program, Department of Psychiatry, University of British Columbia, Vancouver, BC, Canada
Medical Director, Eating Disorders Program, St Paul's Hospital, Vancouver, BC, Canada
British Columbia Provincial Director of Eating Disorders, Vancouver, BC, Canada
Epidemiologist, Centre for Health Evaluation and Outcome Sciences
St Paul's Hospital, Vancouver, BC, Canada

Richard Crawford
Division of Dermatology, University of British Columbia, Vancouver, BC, Canada

Deborah M. Hodgson
Laboratory of Neuroimmunology, School of Behavioural Sciences, University of Newcastle, Callaghan, NSW, Australia

Michael R. Kohn
The Children's Hospital of Westmead, University of Sydney, Sydney, NSW, Australia

Peta Marks
Centre for Mental Health, New South Wales Department of Health, Sydney, NSW, Australia

James E. Mitchell
Neuropsychiatric Research Institute, Fargo, ND, USA

Sue Paxton
Psychology Department, University of Melbourne, Melbourne, VIC, Australia

Jorge Pinzon
British Columbia's Children's Hospital, University of British Columbia, Vancouver, BC, Canada

Christopher Thornton
Carlingford Day Centre, Sydney, NSW, Australia

Ingrid Tyler
St Paul's Hospital Eating Disorders Program, University of British Columbia, Vancouver, BC, Canada

Alison Wakefield
Department of Dietetics, Royal Prince Alfred Hospital, Sydney, NSW, Australia

Abbreviations

AN	anorexia nervosa
APA	American Psychiatric Association
BMI	body mass index (the weight in kilograms divided by the square of the height in meters)
BN	bulimia nervosa
CT	computed tomography
DEXA	dual X-ray absorptiometry
DSM	*Diagnostic and Statistical Manual*
EDNOS	eating disorder not otherwise specified
folate	folic acid
ICD	*International Classification of Diseases*
JVP	jugular venous pressure
MRI	magnetic resonance imaging
PMN	polymorphonuclear leukocyte
QT interval	the time the ventricles (large chambers of the heart) take to recharge
QTc	the QT interval corrected to the patient's heart rate
RBC	red blood cell
TBF	total body fat
WBC	white blood cell
WHO	World Health Organization

Introduction

This book is rather different from most written on eating disorders. Its sole purpose is to provide assistance to health professionals in the understanding, treatment, and management of patients with eating disorders, particularly that part of their treatment that is best described as medical. It is concerned primarily with anorexia nervosa (AN), as this is the member of this group of illnesses that has the most serious medical manifestations, the greatest and longest lasting physical morbidity, and the highest mortality rate. However, relevant issues relating to the other eating or dieting disorders but not obesity, are also discussed.

The intended audience is predominantly medical practitioners, psychiatrists, physicians, pediatricians, and general practitioners – as one of them should always be responsible for the physical health of the eating disorder patient. It is envisaged that this book will also be helpful to other health professionals involved with these patients, particularly nurses, dietitians, and psychologists. The authors intend to produce another book on the same theme but aimed at patients, their families, and carers as well as other stakeholders such as schoolteachers and counselors.

This book is written partly as a reference textbook and partly as a manual for consultation. We suggest that the reader studies Chapters 1–5, leaving the other chapters until the need arises or in order to satisfy that most persistent of intellectual urges, their curiosity. The bibliography found at the back of the book leads the reader to those papers that the authors deem to be the most noteworthy on the various issues surrounding the medical management of eating disorders.

Despite the rather authoritarian and dogmatic format, the principal authors acknowledge the limitations of their expertise. They have between them more than 60 years of experience in treating eating disorder patients. Whatever success they may have had is because they have stood on the shoulders of those who went before them. They trust that discussion and feedback on the book will improve their clinical practice in future.

Eating disorders are orphan conditions: everyone has opinions about them, but no discipline is willing to assume overall responsibility for their care. At one extreme, severe AN with cachexia, multiple nutrient deficiencies, blood and electrolyte abnormalities, and organ dysfunction is a serious physical disease with a chronic course and a high mortality rate. At the other, excessively restricted eating, obligatory exercise, and the occasional use of purging and vomiting are so common in many developed societies, particularly among young women and adolescent girls, as to be almost the norm. In between these extremes are the psychiatric illnesses of moderate anorexia nervosa, bulimia nervosa (BN), atypical or eating disorder not otherwise specified, and perhaps binge eating disorder. These are mental illnesses rather than physical diseases, although they may have serious physical manifestations.

The dichotomy between mental "illness" and physical "disease" implies an acceptance of a dualistic view of body and mind, or soma and psyche. The authors do not wish to endorse or refute this dualism. The opposition of dualism to physicalism was a topic of philosophical debate long before Descartes' influential writings in the fourteenth century, and it should remain so. Health care workers and clinicians are practical persons, and, as such, they are concerned with the practical issues of maintaining health and combating ill health, not with esoteric issues of ultimate reality. From a clinical viewpoint, both the unified and dualistic approaches have advantages. The unified view of body and mind is essential in that almost all of medicine is psychosomatic medicine; psychological factors influence physiological processes and may lead to somatic pathology; physical disease affects the mind both directly and indirectly. Thus, from a psychological perspective, we support a unified concept of body and mind. But in the real world of practice, we recognize that medicine and the health professions involve two complementary approaches: one is concerned with the anatomical structure and physiological processes of the body and their distortions. The other is concerned with the contents of mind, with emotion, and with behaviour and its motivation. The diligent health care worker keeps both in mind but is careful to distinguish in practice between that which requires physical treatment and that which requires psychological care. Perhaps nowhere else in medicine is the failure to make this distinction as disastrous as it is in respect to anorexia nervosa and its related illnesses. And, paradoxically, perhaps nowhere in medicine is it as important to run the two approaches in a complementary fashion. The therapist – or, better, the team of therapists – must be physician, nurse, and dietician, as well as psychiatrist, psychologist, and mental health nurse.

Clinicians treating patients with eating disorders have a complex task. First, they must identify and treat that physical disease that is caused by the dysfunctional behavior and that is manifest in the pathology of malnutrition, chemical disturbance, and organ dysfunction. Next, they must attend to the mental illness that may or may not have some physical basis (we do not know as yet). Third, they must provide help and support in respect to those aspects of these disorders that are best considered as reactions to the dilemma of controlling weight and shape in a society in which obesity has reached epidemic proportions and in which there are strong social pressures to be thinner than most people can achieve.

Good luck to those of you who have chosen to become involved in the management of these demanding patients. Please remember: eating disorders are legitimate illnesses. Those suffering from them deserve the same care and consideration as other sick people.

PART I

The medical perspective

Chapter 1
Definitions and epidemiology

1.1 Nutritional disease and disordered eating

Disordered eating behavior is a common cause of nutritional disorder. The term is used to indicate those instances in which the nutritional disturbance arises from the person's eating behavior rather than from physical or socioeconomic factors. Fasting for religious reasons or as a means of political manipulation are examples of the latter; only rarely do they cause major problems. In many countries, overeating has become the most common form of disordered eating, and its nutritional consequence, obesity, is a major problem area for public health. Disordered eating is not seen as an illness per se, and the response of health workers is to provide nutritional education and to encourage motivation in changing eating practices. Unfortunately, these efforts are often unsuccessful, and insufficient sympathy and assistance are available for those people whose eating is disordered.

Overweight and obesity

Overweight means that weight is higher than "normal," where "normal" may relate to a population norm or to the likelihood of disease. However, the excess weight may be due to excess fluid, muscle, feces, urine, clothing, intra-abdominal fluid, or pregnancy. "Obesity," on the other hand, means there is an excess of body fat. This excess usually results from a combination of increased caloric intake and decreased activity. Obesity is one of the major health problems of the developed world and is becoming much more common in developing nations. An increase in intra-abdominal fat is the primary cause of insulin resistance, which in turn leads to hypertension, high blood fats, diabetes mellitus, and atherosclerosis. The most common medical complications stemming from obesity are listed in Table 1.1.

Table 1.1. *Medical complications of obesity*

Cardiovascular
   Hypertension
   Atherosclerotic cardiovascular disease, including myocardial infarction
   Ventricular hypertrophy and congestive heart failure
   Cerebrovascular accident
Endocrine
   Diabetes mellitus
   Hyperlipidemia
Gastrointestinal
   Gall bladder disease; risk increased further during rapid weight loss
   Fatty liver, portal inflammation, and fibrosis – non-alcoholic steatohepatitis
Metabolic
   Hyperlipidemia, especially hypertriglyceridemia
   Gout
Skeletal
   Degenerative osteoarthritis
   Increased risk of hip fracture
Pulmonary
   Sleep apnea
   Obesity hypoventilation syndrome (Pickwickian syndrome)
Other medical
   Increased cancer risk, especially breast, uterus, colon, prostate
   Increased surgical risk

Obesity is not considered a psychiatric disorder because it is not associated with consistent behavioral and psychological features. However, psychological symptoms such as unhappiness and depression are often present, especially in women. There is a role for mental health input into the support and counseling of obese people, particularly children, before they are caught in a vicious cycle of stigma, decreased physical activity, and alternating overeating and attempted food restriction (dieting). Primary prevention of obesity is paramount because of the limited success of maintaining weight that is lost. Unfortunately, the eating disorder lobby and the obesity lobby may give contradictory messages to health professionals and the general public, one condemning dieting and food restriction and the other promoting them. A balanced approach to promoting healthy eating and exercise is required. Although this text will not focus on obesity, a basic knowledge of obesity helps in the understanding and treatment of patients with eating disorders.

Eating or dieting disorders

Eating disorders refer to those instances of disordered eating that are considered as illnesses because they are associated with a consistent cluster of behavioral and psychological features, imply a predictable course, and are seen by patients, their carers, and health workers as constituting a clinical problem requiring treatment. Because restricted eating, with or without reactive overeating, is involved in most cases, they might better be designated as dieting disorders. Because their characteristics are behavioral and psychological, they are included among psychiatric disorders.

There are two well-recognized syndromes of eating or dieting disorders: anorexia nervosa (AN) and bulimia nervosa (BN). Both are mental disorders included in the *Diagnostic and Statistical Manual* (DSM) IV (1994) and International Classification of Diseases (ICD)-10 (1992) classifications. AN is a disorder of low prevalence, often with a prolonged course, severe medical and psychiatric morbidity, and high mortality. BN is a disorder of rather higher prevalence, with a better prognosis and a shorter course. Both disorders are defined by diagnostic criteria that have changed over time, and this has contributed to difficulty in estimating their frequency.

There is a third category of people with eating disorders who do not fulfill the diagnostic criteria of AN or BN. They are grouped under the heading "atypical eating disorders" or "eating disorders not otherwise specified" (EDNOS). The term refers to a heterogeneous group of problems. It includes people with a milder form of AN or BN (so as to fall short of diagnostic criteria), those who have recovered partially from these illnesses, those who may progress to AN or BN, and truly atypical presentations as with hypochondriasis, mania, depression, and schizophrenia. Significant psychiatric symptomatology may coexist in this group, such as depression, anxiety, obsessionality, and substance misuse. The early identification and intervention of eating disorders involves recognition of people who are still at the atypical or EDNOS stage.

While some people with eating disorders do have nutritional problems as a result of their illness (the under- and malnutrition of AN, the obesity of some atypical eating disorders), others come to medical attention because of the associated psychiatric symptoms or the deleterious effects of specific behaviors, such as vomiting and purging.

Binge eating disorder (BED), which indicates bulimia without compensatory behaviors to prevent weight gain, is more common than AN or BN and is usually included in the EDNOS group. BED is associated with obesity and has a better prognosis than BN. BED may respond to psychological and dietary treatment.

Table 1.2. *Presentation of anorexia nervosa*

Deliberate loss of weight
Extreme reluctance to eat sufficient energy-rich foods to regain and
     maintain a normal, healthy state of nutrition
Characteristic psychopathology
Associated psychiatric symptoms
Associated physical dysfunctions

1.2 Demography and epidemiology

Eating disorders are associated with significant psychosocial and physical disability and impose a heavy burden on the community, particularly in girls and young women aged 15–24 years, where they rank in seriousness with depression, bipolar disorder, alcohol dependence, and harmful substance use. Depending on how strictly diagnostic criteria are applied, eating disorders may be seen either as high-prevalence conditions, usually of only moderate severity, or as low-prevalence conditions of major severity.

Anorexia nervosa

AN is a low-prevalence disorder, often with a prolonged course and with serious physical and psychiatric manifestations (Table 1.2). Females are ten times more likely than males to contract the disorder. The lifetime risk for females is reported variously to be between 0.2% and 0.5%. The figures are comparable with other serious, low-prevalence conditions, such as schizophrenia (lifetime risk of 1.0%) and insulin-dependent diabetes mellitus, which, despite their relatively low prevalence, have a major impact on health and health services because of their chronic course and serious nature.

Psychiatric and physical morbidity are prominent features of AN, which has the highest mortality rate of any psychiatric disorder. Studies of clinic populations have reported consistent findings of outcome and mortality. At five-year follow-up, only 75% of people with AN who have attended specialist clinics are even partially recovered, 20% have become chronic, and 5% have died. At 20-year follow-up, about 80% are recovered, 15% have died, and 5% remain chronic. These levels of chronicity and cumulative mortality indicate the need for long-term continuing care. People with AN are more than 30 times more likely to die as a result of suicide than the general population, and deliberate suicide accounts for more than half of all deaths from AN. Chronic AN confers a degree of disability similar to that of chronic schizophrenia. Milder forms of the illness that do not get to the point of requiring specialist treatment have a far better outcome.

There is a marked gender bias, with more than 90% of cases being female. Despite anecdotal reports, there is no good evidence that the proportion of males is increasing. However, there is evidence that the range of age of onset is becoming wider, with more prepubertal children and older people being affected. Suggested reasons as to why AN is more common in females include physiological mechanisms (the effects of estrogen and zinc on neurotransmitters, and the fact that weight gain and excessive fatty tissue associated with puberty are more prominent in girls) and psychological factors (higher levels of concern about weight and shape and their importance for self-esteem in females). AN is no longer predominantly a disorder of middle-class people, although it may have been so 50 or 100 years ago. In developed societies today, it is distributed fairly evenly between the social classes; it is also found in developing countries.

Diagnostic criteria of anorexia nervosa

The clinical features of AN are easily recognized, and the diagnosis is usually made with high reliability between clinicians. The diagnostic criteria of the two major classificatory systems in current use, DSM IV and ICD-10, are very similar. All of the following signs and symptoms listed in the World Health Organization's (WHO) ICD 10th edition are required for the diagnosis:

- The patient's body mass index (BMI) is 17.5 or less, or body weight is maintained at least 15% below the expected or average body weight for the patient's age and sex. If the patient is prepubertal, then the expected weight gain does not occur during the growth period. (Calculation of BMI is discussed below.)
- Weight loss is self-induced and/or sustained through the avoidance of "fattening" foods and through the utilization of other weight-loss tactics.
- Body image distortion and a morbid dread of fatness, such that the patient imposes an unhealthy and unreasonably low weight threshold on themselves.
- There is evidence of endocrine disorder in the form of amenorrhea among women and loss of sexual desire and potency among men. There may also be elevated levels of growth hormone and cortisol, alterations to the metabolism of thyroid hormone, and abnormal insulin secretion.
- In prepubertal patients, puberty is delayed but is often completed normally after recovery.

Bulimia nervosa

BN is a clearly defined psychiatric disorder of moderate severity and with higher prevalence than AN. Between 1.1% and 4.2% of the population are affected. There is a bias towards females, although this is not as strong as in AN. Adolescent girls and young women are more vulnerable, but males and older females are also affected. It is a cause of major psychiatric morbidity. Depression is often prominent and may be intrinsic to the syndrome or a comorbid diagnosis. It is sometimes associated with various forms of personality disorder, with impulsive, dangerous behavior, and with substance abuse.

Atypical eating disorders or eating disorders not otherwise specified

Atypical eating disorders, or EDNOS, are poorly defined and underresearched. The prevalence of EDNOS has not been determined, but it is generally accepted that it is far more common than either AN or BN. Even a single subcategory of EDNOS, BED, which implies bulimia without compensatory behaviors, has been shown to be more common in women attending primary health care than either of the better-recognized disorders.

Boundary issues

While the boundaries between AN and BN and other eating disorders are defined clearly by the diagnostic criteria of the WHO and the American Psychiatric Association (APA) (see Tables 1.3–1.6), the boundary between atypical eating disorders (EDNOS) and "disordered eating" is unclear. The term "not otherwise specified" is easy to understand, i.e. not meeting criteria for the diagnosis of AN or BN. But when does an eating disorder differ from disordered eating? What makes it an illness, rather than an unhealthy behavior, like cigarette smoking?

How does one distinguish between an eating disorder patient (AN, BN, or EDNOS) and a person whose eating behavior is unusual and unhealthy (disturbed or disordered eating)? Eating disorders differ from disordered eating in that patients complain about their eating and seek help for it. However, this is a fairly dubious distinction, as many young women are secretive about their eating and weight concerns or regard them as "normal" even when they are clearly unhealthy. This confusion leads to the contradictory ways in which eating disorders are portrayed in the lay press. Dieting and weight loss rather than weight maintenance are promoted, especially for young women, although excessive emaciation is recognized as abnormal.

Table 1.3. *International Classification of Diseases (ICD)-10 diagnostic criteria for anorexia nervosa*

Body weight is maintained at least 15% below that expected (either lost or never achieved), or Quetelet's body mass index is 17.5 or less. Prepubertal patients may show failure to make the expected weight gain during the period of growth.

Weight loss is self-induced by avoidance of "fattening foods" and one or more of the following: self-induced vomiting, self-induced purging, excessive exercise, use of appetite suppressants and/or diuretics.

There is body-image distortion in the form of a specific psychopathology, whereby a dread of fatness persists as an intrusive, overvalued idea, and the patient imposes a low weight threshold on themselves.

A widespread endocrine disorder involving the hypothalamic-pituitary-gonadal axis is manifest in women as amenorrhea and in men as a loss of sexual interest and potency. (An apparent exception is the persistence of vaginal bleeds in anorexic women who are receiving replacement hormonal therapy, most commonly taken as a contraceptive pill.) There may also be elevated levels of growth hormone, raised levels of cortisol, changes in the peripheral metabolism of thyroid hormone, and abnormalities of insulin secretion.

If onset is prepubertal, then the sequence of pubertal events is delayed or even arrested (growth ceases; in girls, the breasts do not develop and there is primary amenorrhea; in boys, the genitals remain juvenile). With recovery, puberty is often completed normally, but menarche is late.

Subclinical levels of eating disorders, such as disordered eating, restrained eating, binge eating, fear of fatness, purging, and distortion of body image, are all more common among young people. Children in preschool have negative feelings towards their obese peers. There is evidence to suggest that internalization of the "thin ideal" begins in primary school in girls as young as six years of age, but not so for boys. In boys, the negative feelings towards obesity begin at the same time but they are not internalized. Another difference in boys is that the ideal shape is usually a muscular "V" shape. Secondary-school students, in particular girls, report being overwhelmed by body image and weight issues, considering it something they have grown up with. Constantly worrying about the fat content of food, and the size and shape of their bodies, can contribute to a "normative discontent." It is considered "normal" to be concerned about physical appearance. Adolescent girls are often praised when they take steps to "improve" their appearance. Even in this group of young women with subclinical levels of eating behaviors and concerns of body shape and size, there are high

Table 1.4. *Diagnostic and Statistical Manual (DSM)-IV diagnostic criteria for anorexia nervosa*

Refusal to maintain body weight at or above a minimally normal weight for age and height (e.g. weight loss leading to maintenance of body weight less than 85% of that expected; or failure to make expected weight gain during period of growth, leading to body weight less than 85% of that expected).

Intense fear of gaining weight or becoming fat, even though underweight.

Disturbance in the way in which one's body weight or shape is experienced, undue influence of body weight or shape on self-evaluation, or denial of the seriousness of the current low body weight.

In postmenarcheal females, amenorrhea, i.e. absence of at least three consecutive menstrual cycles. (A woman is considered to have amenorrhea if her periods occur only following hormone, e.g. estrogen, administration.)

Specify type:

Restricting type: during the current episode of anorexia nervosa, the person has not engaged regularly in binge eating or purging behavior (i.e. self-induced vomiting or misuse of laxatives, diuretics, or enemas).

Binge eating/purging type: during the current episode of anorexia nervosa, the person has engaged regularly in binge eating or purging behavior (i.e. self-induced vomiting or misuse of laxatives, diuretics, or enemas).

Table 1.5. *International Classification of Diseases (ICD)-10 diagnostic criteria for bulimia nervosa*

There is a persistent preoccupation with eating and an irresistible craving for food. The patient succumbs to episodes of overeating, in which large amounts of food are consumed in short periods of time.

The patient attempts to counteract the "fattening" effects of food by one or more of the following: self-induced vomiting, purgative abuse, alternating periods of starvation, use of drugs such as appetite suppressants, thyroid preparations, or diuretics. When bulimia occurs in diabetic patients, they may choose to neglect their insulin treatment.

The psychopathology consists of a morbid dread of fatness, and the patient sets themselves a sharply defined weight threshold, well below the premorbid weight that constitutes the optimum or healthy weight in the opinion of the physician. There is often, but not always, a history of an earlier episode of anorexia nervosa, the interval between the two disorders ranging from a few months to several years. This earlier episode may have been expressed fully or may have assumed a minor cryptic form with a moderate loss of weight and/or a transient phase of amenorrhea.

Table 1.6. *Diagnostic and Statistical Manual (DSM)-IV diagnostic criteria for bulimia nervosa*

Recurrent episodes of binge eating. An episode of binge eating is characterized by both of the following:

Eating, in a discrete period of time (e.g. within any two-hour period), an amount of food that is definitely larger than most people would eat during a similar period of time and under similar circumstances.

A sense of lack of control over eating during the episode (e.g. a feeling that one cannot stop eating or control what or how much one is eating).

Recurrent inappropriate compensatory behavior in order to prevent weight gain, such as self-induced vomiting, misuse of laxatives, diuretics, enemas, or other medications, fasting, or excessive exercise.

The binge eating and inappropriate compensatory behaviors both occur, on average, at least twice a week for three months.

Self-evaluation is influenced unduly by body shape and weight.

The disturbance does not occur exclusively during episodes of anorexia nervosa.

Specify type:

Purging type: during the current episode of bulimia nervosa, the person has engaged regularly in self-induced vomiting or the misuse of laxatives, diuretics, or enemas.

Non-purging type: during the current episode of bulimia nervosa, the person has used other inappropriate compensatory behaviors, such as fasting or excessive exercise, but has not engaged regularly in self-induced vomiting or the misuse of laxatives, diuretics, or enemas.

levels of mental and physical distress, such as increased levels of depression and reduced health and nutrition. They too require help and guidance.

1.3 Risk factors

Eating habits and body composition are established in childhood and adolescence. Dieting behaviors and disordered eating reported early in adolescence are generally maintained. Body dissatisfaction predicts dieting, and dieting is a risk factor for developing eating disorders. Although dieting is common, only a relatively small percentage of dieters will develop a diagnosable eating disorder. Thus, prior dieting and extreme dieting are common and perhaps even necessary causes for an eating disorder, but they are not in themselves sufficient

Table 1.7. *Prognostic factors for anorexia nervosa*

Favorable factors	Unfavorable factors
Absence of severe emaciation (i.e. body mass index >17) Absence of serious medical complications Motivation to change present behaviors Presence of supportive family and friends	Presence of vomiting in very malnourished patients, particularly vomiting that has become so frequent as to be almost automatic Later age of onset History of neurotic and personality disturbances Disturbed family relationships Longer duration of illness

to result in an eating disorder unless other risk factors are present. As yet, clear indicators pointing to which individuals with disordered eating will progress to an eating disorder have not been identified, but there are some views about the matter that are held widely.

Reports suggest that there is a significantly increased risk of developing an eating or dieting disorder when there is a family history of eating disorders, family dieting, or adverse comments from family members about eating, appearance, or weight. Other purported risk factors include childhood obesity, parental obesity, early menarche, and exposure to or concurrent presentation of affective disorder, substance abuse, or obsessive-compulsive disorder. There is a strong familial association with these illnesses. Some suggest that there may be a causative genetic component.

1.4 Outcome in anorexia nervosa

Most young people who suffer short-term weight loss are not diagnosed as having AN and are never seen for it. The statistics that follow relate to those who have diagnosed AN that has led them to seek care by a specialized eating disorder program. Of these patients, about half will remain anorexic for more than seven years and about 18% will die within 20 years of the diagnosis being made. About half the deaths from anorexia are caused by suicide and half are due to a medical cause. The medical cause is most often sudden death presumed due to dysrhythmia of the heart. Prognostic factors in the outcome of anorexia nervosa are listed in Table 1.7.

Physical outcome

With recovery from AN, physical health can be regained. Patients can live a long and normal life. Fertility is not impaired, and pregnancy and normal childbirth can be achieved. There is no evidence of permanent brain injury, permanent heart injury, or permanent kidney injury in recovered patients who did not suffer a catastrophic event.

Possible permanent physical complications are loss or erosion of teeth, Korsakoff's syndrome (the permanent clinical syndrome of impaired short-term memory that results if Wernicke's encephalopathy is not treated), and perhaps osteopenia. Whether bone density can return to "normal" is not known, but recovery to "within normal limits" is possible.

The most common long-term symptoms after recovery from AN are those related to the bowel. Constipation, bloating, and abdominal pains may last for decades or even permanently. The most common complaint that endangers health is osteoporosis. Recurrent bone fractures can cause chronic pain and lead to chronic disability.

Those patients who do not recover suffer from progressive weakness, decreased exercise tolerance, bone pains and fractures, episodes of faintness, tiredness, stress incontinence of the bladder, bowel pain, cramping, and bloating, and decreased ability to recover from bacterial infections or for wounds to heal following surgery.

Psychiatric outcome

The recovered AN patient can live a normal life. They can return to work, have families, and chase their dreams. They will, however, always have a greater concern than others about weight and shape, and they are likely to respond to a life trauma with recurrent anorexia behavior.

Patients who are chronically anorexic become reclusive, have low self-esteem, and remain obsessional and depressed. Life is a series of health care and personal episodes that are debilitating to the patient and their loved ones.

Suicide as a result of depression presents the greatest risk in AN. Treatment of depression in AN is complicated by the long-term nature of AN and by the reduced effectiveness of antidepressants in malnutrition.

1.5 Course and outcome of bulimia nervosa and binge eating disorder

Half a dozen studies have reported on the outcome of BN, and a couple have reported on the outcome of BED. Although the findings of these studies were fairly consistent with each other, they were limited by the facts that they were all studies of patients who sought treatment, and only one involved repeated assessment. The recent study of Fairburn and colleagues is the only one that has examined the natural course of these illnesses. They reported their findings in two community-based cohorts, which were studied prospectively over five years. One comprised 102 participants with BN; the other was composed of 48 participants with BED (22% with comorbid obesity).

Both cohorts showed marked initial improvement followed by gradual improvement thereafter. Between one-half and two-thirds of the BN cohort had some form of eating disorder of clinical severity at each 15-month assessment point (atypical or EDNOS), although only a minority continued to meet diagnostic criteria for BN. Each year, about a third remitted and a third relapsed. The outcome of the BED cohort was better, with the proportion with any form of clinical eating disorder declining to 18% by five-year follow-up. The relapse rate was low among this cohort. There was little movement of participants across the two diagnostic categories.

At five-year follow-up, 15% (14 of 92) of the BN cohort still met DSM IV criteria for this disorder. An additional 36% (33 of 92) had some other form of clinical eating disorder (2% AN, 34% EDNOS). Eight percent (7 of 92) met diagnostic criteria for BED. The outcome of the BED group was better, with only 18% having a clinical eating disorder of some form (compared with 51% of the BN cohort). The level of general psychiatric symptoms decreased by an average of 30% in the BN cohort and by 42% in the BED group. The rates of anxiety disorder diagnoses were similar (15% in the BN cohort, 11% in the BED group). Alcohol misuse increased over follow-up in the BN cohort. There was little other drug misuse in either cohort. Self-esteem scores did not change significantly in the BN cohort, whereas they improved in the BED group. There were no significant changes in social adjustment, with the BED cohort continuing to function at a better level.

There was an increase in weight and BMI in both cohorts, with the BN participants gaining on average 3.3 ± 10.1 kg and the BED participants 4.2 ± 9.8 kg.

1.6 Change between diagnostic groups

Patients who present with atypical eating disorders or EDNOS frequently go on to develop either AN or BN. Despite earlier reports to the contrary, a change of diagnosis from AN to BN, or vice versa, is rare. However, within the AN group, movement between the restrictors versus the vomiting and purging subtypes is common.

Chapter 2

The behavioral disorders

2.1 Dieting (restricting) and purging forms of anorexia nervosa

The diagnostic criteria that have been prescribed for AN and the other eating disorders have varied only slightly over the years, and the present form (see Tables 1.3–1.6) is essentially similar to when the disorders were first described. It is important to stress that these descriptions are simply lists of symptoms and signs that are commonly associated and that point to a similarity of course of others. They are not true definitions of an illness entity as is found in many instances elsewhere in medicine, i.e. an explanatory portrayal of etiological factors, pathology and physiopathology, derived manifestations, and a course of progression. Instead, they merely note physical, psychological, and behavioral features without a clear appreciation of their interrelationship. The most characteristic of the features of an eating disorder are the behavioral disturbances that the patient displays; it is these features that will be described here.

Anorexic behaviors, although all directed at either decreasing energy intake or increasing energy expenditure, are not uniform (Table 2.1). Some patients employ only the restrictive behaviors commonly associated with "normal" dieting, such as undereating, refusal of high-energy foods, and strenuous exercise. This is the "dieting" or "restricting" form of the illness; these patients differ from normal mainly in the extent of these behaviors and their inability to desist. Other patients also use vomiting and laxative or diuretic abuse. The presentation, then, is of the "purging" form of AN. The distinctions between the two forms of the illness are important, particularly in respect to prognosis (purging being worse). Unfortunately, the advent of the concept of the less serious illness of BN has obscured the difference between restricting and purging anorexics, the latter often being misdiagnosed as "bulimic."

Table 2.1. *Weight-loss behaviors*

Self-induced vomiting (sometimes with the assistance of emetics such as ipecac)
Self-induced purging (abuse of laxatives or high quantities of fibrous foods, such as unprocessed bran or prunes)
Excessive exercise
Use of appetite suppressants, stimulants, or excessive thyroid hormone
Use of diuretics
Fasting
Sucking and spitting food
Use of enemas or suppositories
Misuse of insulin in diabetics
Self-gavage
Self-phlebotomy

Some of the physical symptoms of AN are related directly to the effects of semi-starvation while other physical symptoms are associated mainly with behavioral problems, such as excessive exercising, vomiting, and purging.

The frequency of the restricting and bingeing – purging subtypes of AN is the same. Anorexics who binge and purge are subject to the medical complications of the restrictive behaviors (predominately undernutrition) and of the "bulimic" behaviors, particularly purging and vomiting.

2.2 Restricting behaviors

Food choices are determined by misconceptions acquired from dubious sources such as popular magazines. As fads have changed over the years, so have the foods that are rejected. In the 1960s, patients selectively avoided simple sugars and other carbohydrates (sweets and potatoes). In the 1980s and 1990s, fatty foods and red meat were considered "unhealthy," and vegetarianism became the most common dietary perversion. Energy-reduced dietary products, foods with high fiber content, and supplementary vitamins are preferred. Further changes in the next decade may include an avoidance of genetically modified foods.

In the early phase of their illness, the anorexic patient chooses a diet that is low in energy-dense foods but relatively high in proteins and other essential nutrients. Dietary protein, together with the high activity levels that are characteristic of the illness, exert a nitrogen-sparing effect, and initial weight loss is due almost entirely to loss of adipose tissue. However, when fat reserves are exhausted, and when food refusal becomes more severe, protein catabolism increases. Water loss is accelerated, leading to metabolic and electrolyte disturbances.

At the table, patients cut their food into minute portions, choose inappropriate utensils (a teaspoon for dessert), eat painfully slowly, add excessive condiments, adopt a bizarre sequence of dishes, drink too much (or too little) fluid, dispose of food secretly, and count calories. These behaviors result in conflict with the family, which, together with the patient's increasing anxiety related to food, lead the patient to avoid eating in company. The patient takes different meals and eats at different times, often late at night after hours of procrastination. Patients become overinvolved in reading recipe books and cooking, and may take over the responsibility of preparing the family meals, although they will eat hardly anything themselves. Other family members, including pets, put on weight, while the patient becomes thinner. Less commonly, the anorexic patient imposes their Spartan diet on the whole family. In small children, one of the reasons for failure to thrive is an anorexic mother. Table 2.2 lists some of the abnormal eating-related behaviors of AN.

2.3 Overactivity

Most AN patients are overactive. This is almost as characteristic as the dietary restriction, and it is just as difficult to modify. There are two kinds of presentation.

First, many patients exercise deliberately to burn calories and induce weight loss. Activity may be surreptitious, such as going up and down stairs frequently on various pretexts, or getting off public transport several stops before the destination and walking the rest of the way. Some quote the phrase: "Never sit if you can stand, never stand if you can walk, never walk if you can run." For others, the activity is strenuous physical exercise, usually in the form of aerobic classes or running. Typically, the exercise is solitary. It has a strongly obsessive character and is performed in a regular and rigid sequence. Patients feel guilty if they do not do the exercise. Exercise and eating are linked by "debting" behavior: the patient "earns" the right to eat by undertaking prescribed activities; conversely, they "pay" for self-indulgence by an extra exercise session.

The second presentation is a persistent restlessness that occurs late in the illness. It is associated with sleep disturbance, beyond the occasional normal

Table 2.2. *Abnormal eating-related behaviors of anorexia nervosa*

Food choice
  Obsessional calorie counting or measurement of food quantities
  Eating different food from the rest of the family
  Excessive water consumption
  Excessive use of condiments (e.g. mustard)
  Unusual or inappropriate combinations of food
  Excessive use of diet foods (e.g. low-fat or artificially sweetened)
  Fussiness about food or claiming to have a dislike of, or a "reaction" to,
    particular foods, especially red meat, sweets, and fatty foods
  Difficulty in choosing what to eat
  Feeling full after eating only a small amount of food

Food manipulation
  Eating extremely slowly
  Cutting food into tiny pieces
  Pushing food around the plate or "playing" with the food
  Secretly disposing of food during meals (e.g. feeding a pet under the
    table, wrapping food in a napkin, or putting food in pockets)
  Eating food in a specific sequence
  Using inappropriate eating utensils
  Excessive handling of food and a desire to do the shopping and take over
    the preparation of meals

Abnormal social behaviors
  Refusal to eat
  Reluctance to eat with other people and minimal conversation during
    meals
  Eating at different times from the rest of the family
  Leaving the table frequently during meals, especially to go to the
    bathroom
  Excessive interest in what others are eating
  Desire to talk about food all the time

awakening for urination, and similar to the ceaseless overactivity seen in laboratory animals when they are deprived of food. Restlessness persists until the patient's physical condition has deteriorated to weakness and lassitude. The overactivity may be related to the fall in core body temperature seen in severely ill anorexia patients. A passage in an early paper by one of the nineteenth-century pioneers in this area, William Gull, emphasizes that warming is as essential as feeding in treating the anorexia patient. The need to raise core body temperature may also account for the paradoxical increase noted in diet-induced thermogenesis in anorexia patients during feeding.

2.4 Purging behaviors

In addition to food restriction, many patients use vomiting, laxatives, and diuretic abuse to further induce weight loss. This purging form of illness is particularly malignant, since the behaviors themselves are injurious to health. Serious physical complications arise in patients who maintain a persistently low weight and in whom purging is prominent.

At first, some physical maneuver is necessary to bring on retching, but patients soon learn to vomit at will. Strong cathartics or herbal laxatives are also taken, ostensibly to combat constipation but really to induce diarrhea. Although patients believe that the diarrhea will prevent them from absorbing calories, the weight loss produced is simply the result of dehydration. Oral diuretics have a similar effect. The misuse of weight-loss medications, stimulants, and thyroid hormone is common.

Compared with "restricting-only" patients, purging anorexics are more likely to have problems with impulse control and substance abuse.

Less common forms of purging are the use of enemas and suppositories, the underuse of insulin in diabetics, self-gavage with a nasogastric tube and syringe, and self-phlebotomy.

2.5 Subjective and objective binges

There is confusion between BN and the serious purging form of AN. Anorexia patients often say they are also bulimic. They mean that they eat more than they would wish, i.e. subjective rather than objective binges. The experience of having lost control of eating is important psychopathologically, but it is different from true or objective gorging. A minority of patients have objective binges. Because being undernourished is more important clinically than having binges, anorexia trumps bulimia in patients who are both emaciated and bulimic (binge-eating). Purging behavior is serious in both sets of patients, but particularly in those who are also undernourished.

Chapter 3

History, examination, and investigations

3.1 Special considerations for history taking in eating disorder patients

Leave your office to meet the patient and observe their behavior with those who have accompanied them. Note their state of affect and ability to walk, then gait, weakness, and unsteadiness.

Certain elements of the history, such as those related to abuse or sexual issues, may best be left to a subsequent interview when rapport has been developed.

Instruct the patient to change in a private area, to keep on their underwear, and to wear the gown open to the back. Examining the patient while fully dressed may lead to failure to observe the degree of emaciation and other physical signs. It is preferable to perform the physical examination in the presence of a female trusted by the patient. *Do not* do rectal, pelvic, or breast examination as part of an eating disorder assessment physical examination.

3.2 Mental status examination

General appearance and behavior

Does the patient appear physically unwell, anxious, or depressed? Is he or she emaciated, or are they wearing clothes that obscure their figure? Is the patient restless? Many anorexic patients are unable to sit still or even sit, even when asked to do so, and continually jiggle their feet.

Speech

Is the patient communicative, or do they answer only briefly and reluctantly. Does the patient set out to justify their reasons for dieting? Do they avoid eye contact when asked potentially confrontational questions about eating, exercise, vomiting, or laxative abuse?

Affect and mood

Affect refers to the immediate emotional response in the interview situation. Mood refers to the underlying emotional theme.

Depression and elation

Mild to moderate depression is so common in eating disorders as to be considered intrinsic to the diagnosis. Elation is usually simulated if present.

Anxiety and phobias

A high level of generalized anxiety is often obvious from the patient's avoidant behavior, restlessness, and discomfort in the interview. Patients often admit to a fear of eating, food, or gaining weight, but these fears do not constitute phobias in the full psychiatric sense of the word.

Obsessions and compulsions

Obsessional ruminations about the need to lose weight, dieting, food, and particularly exercise are common and distressing. These are repetitive and troubling thoughts that the patient tries but is unable to suppress. Compulsions or rituals are complicated patterns of behavior designed to reduce anxiety, e.g. cutting food into minute fragments and shuffling it around the plate. Most rituals of an eating disorder patient are related directly to eating, e.g. avoiding "contamination" by touching food. Sometimes, rituals of purification are also found.

Thought

The excessive salience that patients give to ideas of weight, shape, and eating, the need for strenuous exercise, and the importance of abstinence are best considered as overvalued ideas (short of delusions). Eventually, these ideas become so entrenched and resistant to change, despite evidence of serious deterioration of health, and so egocentric that they resemble delusional thinking.

Perception

A distorted image of self by which patients see themselves as obese when emaciated is often cited but is relatively rare in practice. More commonly, patients deny the severity of their weight loss, or say they "feel fat" even though they know that they are not.

Cognition

With increasing debilitation, cognitive function is increasingly impaired. This can progress to confusion and even coma.

Judgment and insight

Judgment and insight of the patient into their illness are characteristically poor, with little appreciation of the seriousness.

Rapport

Patients are often resentful when asked about their symptoms. This is because the condition is often egosyntonic (seen as agreeable) and the patient is often in denial. Previous conflicts with parents or other relatives may lead patients to become especially sensitive about all matters concerning their illness. To establish rapport, it is necessary to show an interest in the patient as a person, and their own perception of the situation, rather than to imply that they are being considered merely as a case of an eating disorder.

The reader is referred to Part II for a more comprehensive discussion of the psychiatric and psychological features of eating disorders.

3.3 History taking

Figure 3.1 presents a schema for history recording.

3.4 Physical examination

The usual physical examination should be undertaken at first presentation of the patient, and repeated subsequently as indicated by physical progress. Table 3.1 provides an outline of the physical examination.

Plates 1–11 demonstrate common or important physical findings.

3.5 Methods of measuring body weight and body fat

Table 3.2 summarizes the benefits and limitations of the commonly used methods of measuring body weight and body fat. In most clinical settings, BMI will

Identifying information
Name
Date of birth
Address
Work phone number
Home phone number
Permission to contact and any special instructions

Permission to contact: to protect confidentiality, obtain specifics of where you may contact them (who, where, how?)

Referral source
Date of examination

History of present illness
Indicate what history is obtained from collateral sources and from whom, both medical and psychiatric

Weight

At 5–10 years	Maximum weight	Desired weight
Early in teens	Usual weight	Preferred weight
Later in teens	Lowest weight	Healthiest weight
Adult weight	Wish for weight change	
Periods of weight loss		
Attitudes about shape and size		
Feelings about size and shape		

Weight: there is usually a difference between the weight the patient believes would be medically acceptable and that which they would find acceptable

Eating behavior

Eating: average day now	Breakfast	Snack	Lunch	Snack	Dinner	Snack

List of foods they will eat
List of foods they will not eat
Food allergies/intolerances: what food and what happens?
Vegetarian? Vegan?
Intolerances (e.g. lactose)
Preferences
Religious and cultural beliefs
Time course of beliefs about food
Beliefs about food composition

Figure 3.1. Schema for medical history taking for patients with eating disorders.

Adaptive behaviors

Exercise
Current pattern of exercise
Types of exercising (aerobic/anaerobic)
Most extreme exercise
Duration of exercise per 24 hours
Is exercise obligatory?
Effects of missing a day of exercise
Debit (e.g. what food would they not eat?)

Purging
Fluid loading
Purge
How long after binge?
How?
Times vomited
Blood vomited   How often?   How much?
Use of (what, how much, when?):
   Laxatives, enemas, suppositories
   Diuretics, ipecac, fasting, exercise
   Misuse of insulin, self-phlebotomy, self-gavage

*Purging behaviors: take a history of all the purging behaviors that have
   been used, not just at present*

Binge eating

Binge eating			
First binged	When?	Why?	Where?
Usual binge	What?	Times normal meal	
Ever binge with others?			
Feelings during binge			
Length of binge		Why binge is stopped	Feelings afterwards

Physical symptoms

Head and neck
Hair: loss, new growth
Vision: night, loss of focus

Skin	Dry	Bruising	Rash

Cardiovascular/respiratory

Cardiovascular/respiratory			
Shortness of breath	Orthopnea	Paroxysmal nocturnal dyspnea	Exercise tolerance
Palpitations	Sudden onset/finish	Frequency	Duration

Figure 3.1. (cont.)

	Change recently?	Related to binge and purge?	Rapid or slow rate?
	Regular or irregular?		
Chest pain	Where?	Precipitating factors	Radiation
	Associated symptoms	Description (knife, ache, burning, heaviness, etc.)	Duration?
	Relieving factors		

Sexual and reproductive/menstrual history

Frequency	Periodicity	Flow	Amenorrhea
Oral contraceptives	Anovulation	Pregnancy	Mothering

Urinary

Incontinence	Stress	Volume	
Nocturia	Urinary frequency and volume		

Musculoskeletal

Strength	Weakness (where?)	Cramps (where?, when?)	Numbness
Pains (describe)			

Neurological

Dizziness (describe)	When?	Concentration	Memory

Psychosocial
Depression
Suicidal ideation
Effect of eating disorder on life
Amount of time spent thinking about weight, eating, eating concerns?
Can they eat in front of others?   Who?

Past medical history

Personal history
Allergies to medications and other allergies:
Medications: what?, how much?, do they purge them?, can they take them?
Over-the-counter medications   Illicit drug-taking Cigarettes (how many?, how long?)
Alcohol: wine, beer, hard liquor? How much?
Binge drinking?   The use of alcohol to manage feelings or behaviors?

Figure 3.1. (cont.)

*Smoking is an anorexic behavior (10 calories of energy are burned
    per cigarette)*

Family history

Functional inquiry

Figure 3.1. (cont.)

be measured to follow the patient's response to refeeding. We therefore review
the steps required to obtain the BMI in detail.

Measuring height

- Measure the height with the patient standing, using a stadiometer or portable anthropometer.
- Shoes or socks should not be worn.
- Clothing that allows the patient's posture to be seen should be worn.
- The back and head should be straight and the patient's eyes looking forward.
- Feet, knees, buttocks, and shoulder blades should be in contact with the vertical surface of the stadiometer, anthropometer, or wall.
- Arms should be hanging loosely at the sides, with palms facing the thighs.
- The patient should take a deep breath and stand tall to help straighten the spine.
- The movable headpiece should be lowered gently until it just touches the crown of the head.
- Read the height in meters.

Measuring weight

- Use the same scale each time (preferably one with sliding weights along the top (balance beam scale), as used in hospitals and gymnasiums, since these scales are the most accurate).
- Ensure the scales are calibrated accurately at zero before use.
- Measure the weight before a meal.
- The balance should be placed on a hard, flat surface and zeroed before each measurement.
- The patient should stand unassisted, as still as possible, in the middle of the platform.

Table 3.1. *Schema for the physical examination of patients*
with eating disorders

General inspection	Clothing: disguise, bulky clothing to hide figure, blatant underdressing to display emaciation or for cold exposure

Vital signs
Temperature (ear/mouth/
  axillary/other)
Blood pressure (appropriate
  cuff size)
Right, left
Sitting
Standing
Lying
Respiratory rate
	Always measure the blood pressure and its associated heart rate. Take blood pressure and heart rate in at least one arm with the patient lying down and standing.
	If there is a greater than 10 mm Hg drop in diastolic blood pressure, or 10 beats per minute increase in heart rate, redo the blood pressure and heart rate every 15 seconds until it stabilizes

Head and neck Hair (alopecia)	The most common cause of alopecia is hair loss due to malnutrition. It is a generalized loss of scalp hair, with no signs of inflammation or abnormality of the hair follicle
Eyes (lateral nystagmus) Teeth (erosion) Gums (recession, friable)	With Wernicke's encephalopathy, the most common gaze abnormality is lateral nystagmus (on lateral gaze, the eye moves rapidly back and forth)

Parotid hypertrophy
Submandibular gland
  hypertrophy
Thyroid (normal, enlarged,
  nodule)
	With vomiting, the parotid and submandibular glands are swollen bilaterally. This can also occur with malnutrition alone, although the swelling is usually less marked. The glands are not swollen on one side of the body only

Cardiorespiratory Chest Heart sounds (mid-systolic clicks/murmur) Irregular rhythm Jugular venous pressure	
Abdominal Abdomen (stool/liver/ spleen/mass)	An abdominal mass that can be indented is always stool

(cont.)

Table 3.1. (cont.)

Skin

Skin (dryness, peeling of skin of hands and feet) Hypercarotenemia Acrocyanosis Lanugo hair	Acrocyanosis describes extremities that are constantly a blue color. This is usually due to slow movement of blood. This allows for greater extraction of oxygen from the blood, leading to desaturation of the blood and resulting in cyanosis. Raynaud's phenomenon is no more common in AN than in normals. Raynaud's means that there are phases of color change of the extremities. They may turn one, two, or three of the colors white, purple, and deep red, in that order
Areas of hyperpigmentation Russell's sign	Hyperpigmentation over an area of the trunk can be caused by repeated exposure to heat. This is called erythema ab igne. It occurs due to the attempt of the patient to warm themselves by external warming devices (e.g. hot water bottle or radiator)
Clubbing Self-injury signs (burn or slash marks, raccoon eyes, hair loss, bruises, needle tracks)	Clubbing is not known to be caused by AN, although the authors have seen it in patients with AN without another identifiable cause. The presence of clubbing should prompt a search for a specific cause, e.g. inflammatory bowel disease, Grave's disease, or celiac disease

Neurological

Muscle strength Sensation (touch, joint position sense, temperature sense) Reflexes (delayed relaxation phase of ankle jerk)	Proximal weakness is due to a myopathy. It can be due to potassium, magnesium, phosphate or calcium deficiencies
Chvostek's sign	Chvostek's sign is the involuntary contraction of the seventh cranial nerve caused by tapping over it, where it passes through the parotid gland in front of the ear

(cont.)

Table 3.1. (cont.)

Trousseau's sign	Trousseau's sign is the involuntary contraction of the hand caused by cutting off blood flow to the hand and arm by elevating the pressure in a blood pressure cuff fastened around the arm, above the systolic pressure and waiting, until the hand goes into spasm or discomfort occurs (maximum five minutes)
Lateral peroneal nerve tap sign	The lateral peroneal nerve tap sign is the involuntary dorsiflexion of the foot caused by tapping on the lateral peroneal nerve where it crosses the neck of the fibula

- Occasionally, some patients with AN may try to make themselves appear heavier than they really are by strapping weights close to their body, or by carrying heavy objects in their pockets, or by drinking excessive amounts of water and avoiding urinating before weighing. If possible, for purposes of accurately comparing repeated weights, the weight should be obtained at the same time each day, preferably in the morning, immediately after voiding. Excess clothing, such as coats, scarves, shoes, belts, and watches, should be removed.
- Read the weight in kilograms.

Calculating body mass index

The BMI is the most convenient way to measure the extent to which a patient is underweight or overweight. The BMI can be calculated by dividing the patient's weight in kilograms by the square of their height in meters, as indicated by the following formula:

$$\text{BMI} = \frac{\text{weight}}{(\text{height})^2}$$

where weight is measured in kilograms and height in meters. The use of BMI is recommended because of its convenience, but it has several limitations:

- It is difficult to apply in young children who are growing and whose height may be stunted by the illness.
- It gives no indication of body composition. For example, an athlete may be in the normal BMI range but have extremely low body fat.

Table 3.2. *Methods of measuring body weight*

Test	Tool	Weight	Body fat	Lean mass	Reliability	Limitations	Cost	Availability
Anthropometrics	Skin-fold calipers	No	Yes	No	Low to high	Very observer-dependent	Low	Limited
BMI	Scale	Yes	No	No	High	Does not measure body compartments	Low	Very
DEXA	DEXA machine	No	Yes	Yes	High	Expensive, radiation exposure	High	Limited
CT scan of whole body	CT scanner	No	Yes	Yes	High	Cost, radiation exposure	Very high	Limited
BIA	BIA machine	No	Yes	Yes	Low	Result highly dependent on body water	Moderate	Limited

BIA, biolectrical independence analysis; BMI, body mass index; CT, computed tomography; DEXA, dual X-ray absorptiometry.

- The use of BMI percentiles: because percentiles of BMI are much tighter in children, younger adolescents, and short people, a change in the percentile is a more accurate indicator of undernutrition than BMI itself.
- Body composition by anthropometry: this is potentially a very accurate, reliable, and inexpensive way of estimating total body fat. An experienced colleague can provide the training required. However, without training and experience, the measurements are unreliable. The most important factors to learn are how to determine the sites where measurements should be taken and how much skin and subcutaneous tissue should be "pinched" and measured (not the muscle beneath and not just the skin).

Estimating total body fat using anthropometrics measurements

- Take all measurements on the left side of the body.
- Measure the mid-arm circumference, biceps, and triceps skin fold with the arm held straight forward and parallel to the ground and with the forearm bent straight up at 90 degrees.
- Measure the subscapular and suprailiac skin folds with the arm held loosely at the sides and the shoulders relaxed.
- Midarm point: mark the midarm point by halving the distance measured between the olecranon and the acromion.
- Midarm circumference: at the midarm point, measure the circumference of the arm with the muscles relaxed.
- When using the calipers to measure skin folds, pick up the skin and subcutaneous tissue (subcutaneous fat). Take care not to pick up the underlying muscle or just the skin.
- The biceps skin fold should be measured with the calipers pointing vertically downward, at the midarm point.
- The triceps skin fold should be measured at the midarm point, with the calipers pointing vertically upward from below the arm.
- The subscapular skin fold should be measured at the tip of the scapula, with the calipers held horizontally.
- The suprailiac skin fold should be measured just medial to the anterior superior iliac crest, with the calipers held horizontally.

Body composition by electrical impedence

Various commercial devices are available to estimate body fat by means of passing an electrical current between two specified points on the body surface (flow affected by extent of subcutaneous fat). Unfortunately, this method of measurement is unreliable in patients with disturbed hydration, as is common in eating disorders.

3.6 Routine laboratory testing

Electrolytes and minerals

Bicarbonate (serum)

This is usually normal. It is decreased in acidosis, usually due to starvation ketosis. It is elevated by a hypokalemic metabolic alkalosis due to volume depletion.

Calcium (serum)

The serum calcium is usually normal. Low serum calcium is usually due to low total body magnesium, since magnesium is necessary for the maintenance of serum calcium levels. Low serum calcium may also be due to low serum albumen because calcium is bound to albumen for transport. Measure ionized calcium to determine whether the free calcium in the blood is low.

Magnesium (serum)

Magnesium deficiency in AN is common. Magnesium deficiency results in proximal myopathy, muscle cramping, loss of visual acuity after focusing on a close object (reading) for about 30 minutes, impaired short-term memory, Trousseau's sign, Chvostek's sign, or the lateral peroneal nerve tap sign. More than 99% of magnesium is intracellular. Body stores are usually very low before the serum level drops below normal. Therefore, a low serum level always indicates deficiency, but a normal level does not exclude deficiency. Normal serum magnesium with symptoms or signs of hypomagnesemia is an indication for a magnesium load test to confirm the diagnosis of a total body deficiency.

Phosphorus (serum)

Phosphorus is abundant in food, is easily absorbed from the gut, and moves quickly intracellular along with glucose after meals. Thus, the serum phosphorus level often falls slightly below normal following meals. Phosphorus deficiency is life-threatening because phosphate is necessary for adenosine triphosphate (ATP), cyclic adenosine monophosphate (AMP), 2,3-diphosphoglycerol (2,3-DPG), and many other metabolic processes. Phosphate deficiency can cause congestive heart failure, an organic brain syndrome, rhabdomyolysis, hemolytic anemia, and the dysfunction of all metabolically active organs in the body. The metabolic complications of hypophosphatemia usually have an onset once the serum phosphate falls to less than one-half of the lower limit of normal in an ill patient, or less than one-third the lower limit of normal in a healthy patient. Serum levels drop rapidly in malnutrition. Any fall in phosphorus must be treated urgently.

Potassium (serum)

Serum potassium is commonly low in AN due to loss by vomiting, diuretics or laxatives abuse, or renal loss due to exchange for sodium in volume dehydration.

Sodium (serum)

This is usually normal. The most common abnormality is low serum sodium due to the retention of free water in a purging patient. This is because the body regulates volume as a greater priority than osmolality. Serum sodium may be very low in psychogenic polydipsia, which may accompany AN, in Addison's disease (where it is usually associated with a higher than normal potassium level), in hypothyroidism, in renal failure, and in the face of diuretic use because diuretics decrease the ability of the kidney to regulate sodium balance.

Zinc (serum)

The serum zinc level is an unreliable measure of total body zinc. Most zinc is intracellular. Zinc is bound in the blood to zinc-binding globulin and albumen. Zinc status can be assessed by taste sensation, e.g. with the Accusens T-test. However, taste testing is cumbersome and unreliable. Zinc deficiency is best diagnosed by a dietary history of low zinc intake (ingested zinc comes mostly from milk products and seafood) combined with symptoms of dysgeusia (altered taste sensation) or dry skin, especially desquamating dry skin on the palms and soles.

Blood picture

Complete blood count: hemoglobin, white blood cells, and platelet estimation

Significant malnutrition usually results in a mild normochromic normocytic anemia. However, hemoglobin should not fall below 10 g/l. A hemoglobin level of less than 10 g/l is usually caused by diet-induced iron deficiency, but it may be due to gastrointestinal blood loss, vitamin B12 deficiency, folic acid deficiency, or copper deficiency.

Folate (red blood cell folate)

Green vegetables form the main source of folic acid (folate). Folic acid deficiency may be seen at presentation. More important is refeeding-induced folate deficiency, as this often goes undetected and will limit cell growth and division. Deficiency of folate causes tiredness due to megaloblastic anemia.

Ferritin

Iron deficiency is very common in AN. The chief dietary source of iron is red meat, which is usually avoided by patients with eating disorders. Menstruation, if present, also causes iron loss. Iron deficiency results in tiredness due to associated anemia. Iron deficiency can also change taste and eating behavior. The syndrome of pica, seen in some patients with iron deficiency, results in unusual cravings for food. The commonest form of pica is pagophagia, the craving for ice and very cold liquids. Pica can even result in the craving for dirt or paint.

Other serological parameters

Alkaline phosphatase

Alkaline phosphatase is an enzyme found in bone and the cells lining the ducts within the liver (Kupffer cells). Serum levels are elevated when there is an obstruction to the ductal system of the liver or increased bone formation. Even a single small obstruction in the liver can result in a significant rise in alkaline phosphatase, so the degree of elevation is a poor measure of the degree of abnormality. To determine whether an elevation originates in the liver or bone, order a gamma glutaryl transaminase (GGT) test, since GGT is only released by the liver. If the GGT is elevated, then the alkaline phosphatase elevation is due to liver disease.

Serum aspartate transaminase

Aspartate transaminase (AST) is released from the liver parenchymal cells (hepatocytes) when they are damaged. The serum level in an individual is very constant over time. Elevation of AST is caused by liver damage; it is also caused by muscle damage, as AST is found in muscle as well. The elevation of AST is influenced by the amount of damage and the number of cells that are damaged. Less liver tissue (e.g. in cirrhosis) will lead to a smaller rise in AST for a given injury. To determine whether increased AST is due to liver or muscle injury, a creatine phosphokinase (CPK) test can be ordered. CPK comes from muscle, not liver. An elevation of GGT or nucleotidase (NTD) is specific for liver.

Vitamin B12

Vitamin B12 is usually normal in AN, but it may be low. The serum B12 assay may be falsely low, normal, or high due to measurement error. This occurs occasionally due to a faulty measurement kit. A low vitamin B12 is usually caused by nutritional deficiency in AN. It is due to malabsorption of B12 about 3% of the time. The Schilling's test can be ordered to determine whether B12 deficiency is due to lack of instrinsic factor in the stomach, disease of the ileum, or decreased intake.

Creatine phosphokinase

Elevation of CPK indicates muscle (smooth or striated) damage. In AN without muscle injury, CPK should be low due to reduced muscle mass.

Creatinine (serum)

Creatinine should be in the low range of normal, because the level of creatinine in the blood is proportional to the total body muscle mass. An increase in serum creatinine, even within the normal range, may indicate renal dysfunction. Increased muscle breakdown may result in a slight increase in CPK. The most common cause of renal dysfunction in AN is volume depletion. Other causes include renal stones, infection, urinary tract obstruction due to impaired emptying of the bladder secondary to constipation, autonomic dysfunction, pelvic muscle weakness, and medications.

Thyroid-stimulating hormone

Order the thyroid-stimulating hormone (TSH) test to rule out hyperthyroidism. The TSH assay is very reliable and sensitive, and it is the best single measure of thyroid function, usually obviating the need for other screening tests. Release of thyrotropin-releasing hormone (TRH) from the hypothalamus stimulates the release of TSH from the pituitary gland, which in turn stimulates the thyroid gland itself to release the thyroid hormones thyroxine (T4) and tri-iodothyronine (T3). TSH is elevated in hypothyroidism, as the body attempts to stimulate thyroid hormone production by the thyroid. TSH is low when the thyroid is overactive or with the administration of thyroid hormone.

Note: sick euthyroidism (also known as euthyroid sick syndrome) is very common in AN. It is not hypothroidism. It is an adaptive state. It should not be treated with thyroid hormone.

Urinalysis

Urinalysis is usually normal. Blood in the urine may indicate renal stones. White blood cells in the urine usually indicate infection, which is made more likely if there is dysfunction of bladder emptying secondary to weakness of the pelvic muscles, autonomic dysfunction of the bladder, medications, or the AN itself. Protein in the urine is elevated with strenuous exercise, which is often occult in AN. Elevated urine protein may indicate renal damage.

3.7 Other tests that may be helpful in some patients

Electrocardiogram

The most common finding on electrocardiogram (EKG) is a slow heart rate (bradycardia). This is normal with long-term aerobic training, but it may also be due to malnutrition, hypothyroidism, or the sick euthyroid syndrome seen in severe AN. The period needed for the ventricular muscle to electrically recharge (repolarize; called the QT interval) is adjusted for heart rate to calculate the corrected QT interval (QTc). A correction is used because the time for repolarization is normally longer with a slower heart rate. A prolonged QTc is associated with an increased risk for ventricular dysrhythmia and death. An increase in the QTc by more than 60 ms, or a QTc greater than 450 ms, indicates an increased risk of dysrhythmia. The QT interval can be prolonged by certain medications and medication interactions that involve the cytochrome P450 system.

Chest X-ray

Order in the presence of specific respiratory symptoms, such as shortness of breath, cough, and chest pain. Opacification on the chest X-ray is usually due to aspiration pneumonia. Impaired consciousness and use of a nasogastric tube increase the likelihood of aspiration of gastric contents.

Echocardiogram

This can determine ventricular wall thickness and the cause of a cardiac murmur. It is not sensitive to the presence of mild to moderate mitral valve prolapse when performed in quiet respiration while supine (this is normal for the echocardiogram).

Holter monitor with spectral analysis

The 24-hour or 48-hour Holter monitor captures an EKG recording to assess dysrhythmias, changes consistent with ischemia, and changes in heart rate. In AN, the Holter monitor can help to determine the cause of palpitations on history or dysrhythmia on examination. Spectral analysis is a computer analysis of the Holter record that determines the degree of autonomic dysfunction through heart rate variability.

Pelvic ultrasound

This may be used to visualize ovarian follicles. Ovarian follicles demonstrate that normal endocrine function has returned, an indication that a physiologic body fat has been reached.

Upper gastrointestinal endoscopy

This may be ordered for severe reflux, dysphagia, persistent odynophagia, hematemesis of dark blood, or more than a fleck of bright red blood.

Of course, many of these tests and procedures are troubled by various limitations, such as low reliability, modest utility for certain conditions, low availability, and high cost. These limitations are reviewed in Table 3.3.

3.8 Differential diagnosis of eating disorders

In the absence of behavioral or cognitive indicators of AN, the clinician may suspect a somatic cause of weight loss, such as diabetes mellitus, hyperthyroidism, Addison's disease, human immunodeficiency virus (HIV)/acquired immune deficiency syndrome (AIDS), chronic infectious disease, carcinoma, a malabsorption syndrome (e.g. Sprue), Crohn's disease, or another chronic debilitating disease. However, it is not advisable to encourage extensive and invasive medical investigations if the patient's symptoms can be explained adequately by the diagnosis of AN or another eating disorder.

The physical signs that help to confirm the diagnosis of an eating disorder are Russell's sign, erosion of the teeth, parotid and submandibular gland hypertrophy, hypercarotenemia, lanugo hair, and erythema ab igne.

People who are experiencing a major depressive episode may lose weight coincidentally with the loss of appetite or motivation to eat. However, people with AN do not experience a loss of appetite; rather, they *choose* not to

Table 3.3. *Diagnostic testing: dangers and limitations*

Test	Measures	Primary indication	Limitations	Danger	Cost
BMI	Change in weight corrected to height	To measure the success of feeding	Does not measure whether the change in weight is due to a change in fat, muscle, water, constipation, etc.	None	Low
Anthropometrics	Total body fat	To measure the success of feeding	Reliability of the test is very low unless performed by an experienced observer	None	Low
EKG	Electrical activity of the heart	To measure QT interval, heart rate, heart rhythm	Only takes a 20s record Unlikely to capture an intermittent problem	None	Low
Echocardiogram	Size, shape, and contraction of the heart, as well as valve function	To determine the cause of many heart murmurs, the thickness of the muscle of the heart, and its contractile function	Does not measure electrical activity and is insensitive to certain heart conditions, e.g. mitral valve prolapse	None	Moderate

(cont.)

Table 3.3. (cont.)

Test	Measures	Primary indication	Limitations	Danger	Cost
Holter monitor	Electrical activity of the heart for 24 or 48 hours on one lead	Helps to determine the cause of palpitations, faints due to dysrhythmias, and the degree of autonomic dysfunction	Does not use all of the standard heart leads, so not all parts of the heart will be assessed. Does not assess the anatomy or physical function of the heart	None	Moderate
Chest X-ray	Gross anatomy of the chest and upper abdomen	Helps to determine the cause of shortness of breath and the location of a nasogastric tube placed for feeding	Does not measure lung function. Aspiration may not show up for up to 24 hours The nasogastric tube can move after the X-ray is taken	Low	Low
CT head	Structure of the brain	Differential diagnosis of loss of consciousness or seizures	Does not measure function	Low	High
CT abdomen	Anatomy of the intra-abdominal organs	To rule out superior mesenteric artery syndrome	Does not look into functional causes or microanatomy of abdominal complaints	Low	High

(cont.)

Table 3.3. (cont.)

Test	Measures	Primary indication	Limitations	Danger	Cost
MRI head	Anatomy of brain	Best current technique to image anatomy of the brain	Does not look at brain function Not as readily available as CT	Low	Very high
Functional MRI	Anatomy and some functionality of the brain	May be as good as PET for measuring brain function	Unknown	Low	Very high
PET scan of brain	Function of brain	To determine functional brain abnormalities	Very expensive and not generally available	Low	Very high
Gastric emptying by nuclear medicine	Time taken by the stomach to empty	Differential diagnosis of early satiety and upper abdominal pain	Does not show anatomy of bowel	Low	Moderate
Upper gastrointestinal endoscopy	Appearance of the esophagus, stomach, and part way down the duodenum	Differential diagnosis of dysphagia, odynophagia, early satiety, abdominal pain, and hematochezia	Does not measure contraction of bowel or rule out superior mesenteric artery syndrome	Moderate	High

BMI, body mass index; CT, computed tomography; EKG, electrocardiogram; MRI, magnetic resonance imaging; PET, positron-emission tomography.

eat despite great hunger and desire for food (although they may deny being hungry if asked). Also, unlike people with AN, depressed people do not exhibit an excessive concern about their body shape or the caloric content of food, unless the depression is secondary to a diagnosis of AN or BN. Furthermore, unlike those who are depressed, people with AN will be pleased about their weight loss.

Obsessional symptoms (e.g. fear of eating contaminated food, or decreased food intake due to the urge to chew each mouthful a specific number of times) may also account for weight loss. As always, a thorough psychiatric history will need to be taken before making a firm diagnosis.

Disturbances of eating can occur in association with other disorders. Anorexia and hypophagia are seen in many physical disorders as well as in depression and dementia and sometimes occur in the context of severe personality disturbance. Hyperphagia is characteristic of certain organic disorders, including hypothalamic tumors and the Klein–Levin and Prader–Willi syndromes. Anxiety about eating with others may be an expression of social phobia, and repeated spontaneous vomiting may also be anxiety-related. Such disturbances of eating are not "eating disorders" as such, since they are secondary either to a general medical disorder or to another psychiatric condition.

There is no laboratory test to diagnose eating disorders; neither should the diagnosis be made by exclusion of other diagnoses alone. The diagnosis is best confirmed by identifying cognitions and behaviors.

If, during assessment, the patient denies all symptoms of an eating disorder, then further information may be obtained through:

- Collateral history (as with alcohol abuse, reports by a relative that the patient has AN should never be dismissed without careful checking).
- Observation of the patient in a controlled setting.
- Employing questions that actively challenge cognitions. For example, the following questions may be put to the patient:

  - *Question:* picture yourself at a large buffet dinner that has sliced raw vegetables, potato salad, fruit, bread and rolls of different kinds, sliced ham and beef, sauces and gravies, pies, and cake. What would you eat?
  - *Response:* if the patient is keeping their history covert, they will start off by saying that they would be pleased to eat at the buffet and would help themselves. When pressured to answer what they would eat, they may say, "Some vegetables, perhaps a roll . . ." They may reveal their aversion to fatty and high-calorie foods.
  - *Question:* you have lost 10 kg. If I could wave a magic wand and instantly put 10 kg of fat on your body, would that be all right?

Table 3.4. *Laboratory investigations that are expected to be normal in eating disorders*

Hematological	Clotting indices, platetet count
Biochemistry	Alkaline phosphatase, GGT, bilirubin
Immunological	ANA, RF, ENA, ESR, Schirmer test
Gastrointestinal	D-xylose test, C-14 breath test
Neurological	EEG, MRI head
Endocrine	Prolactin, ACTH stimulation test, TRH stimulation test, anti-thyroid antibodies
Radiological	Skull X-ray, chest X-ray, abdominal X-ray, ultrasound of the abdomen

ACTH, adrenocorticotrophic hormone; ANA, antinuclear antibody; EEG, electroencephalogram; ENA, extractwide nuclear antibody; ESR, erythrocyte sedimentation rate; GGT, gamma glutamyltransferase; MRI, magnetic resonance imaging; RF, rheumatoid factor; TRH, thyrotropin-releasing hormone.

- *Response:* it would be alright ... but it would, of course, have to be muscle, and it would have to go on slowly ... to be healthy (with a look of horror on their face).

• There are a number of laboratory tests that should be normal in AN, BN, and EDNOS (Table 3.4). If they are abnormal, then another disease process may be present.

Ruling out diseases that can mimic eating disorders

Addison's disease

Addison's disease usually presents with weight loss, lethargy, slightly elevated potassium, and slightly low serum sodium. The cortrysn stimulation test (adrenocorticotrophic hormone (ACTH) stimulation test) should be performed to exclude suspected Addison's disease. A doubling of the baseline serum cortisol or a peak serum cortisol of more than 500 IU indicates normal adrenal function and excludes Addison's disease. Glucocorticoid use, other than dexamethasone, will interfere with test results.

Malabsorption

The best test to exclude malabsorption is the fecal fat test. One hundred grams of fat is ingested daily for six days, with stools collected on the last three days. Adults normally absorb more than 95% of the ingested fat. However, this test is usually impossible for an eating disorder patient to undertake due to the requirement to eat a large amount of fat. The test can be performed in the same way with 50 g of fat a day. The D-xylose test may be used to screen for small bowel malabsorption. Small bowel malabsorption or rapid transit will reduce D-xylose absorption.

Hyperthyroidism

The serum TSH will be very low in hyperthyroidism. Hyperthyroidism causes rapid transit in the bowel and can cause malabsorption.

Inflammatory bowel disease

Crohn's disease in teenagers may be associated with anorexia, lethargy, and a depressed mood, sometimes with few gastrointestinal symptoms. Consultation by a gastroenterologist, who will likely perform an endoscopy, is needed to investigate.

Celiac disease

Celiac disease may be very mild and present with weight loss but little or no diarrhea. Tissue transglutaminase antibody is a very sensitive and specific blood test that can help in the diagnosis of celiac disease (sprue).

Chapter 4

Medical manifestations by system

The medical symptoms and signs of AN and, although less serious, of other eating disorders are part of the illness, and hence it is more appropriate to think of them as medical manifestations rather than merely complications. Although the disorder usually starts in adolescence, its course is often prolonged; AN patients may be ill for many years, and the majority of severely ill AN patients are in early or mid adult life. Hence, AN is a matter of concern for adult physicians as well as for pediatricians and adolescent medicine specialists. Figure 4.1 shows a mnemonic that is useful for remembering the physical signs of eating disorders.

Manifestations result from starvation or from the behaviors adopted to induce it. They are not indicative of underlying pathology. The inexperienced clinician who undertakes unnecessary investigations to exclude all possible causes for each abnormal finding is doing the patient a disservice by delaying appropriate treatment. Rather, all clinicians should be aware of the wide range of physical abnormalities that are commonly found in anorexic patients (Table 4.1). Many of these abnormalities, such as decreased serum concentrations of gonadotropins and steroid sex hormones, alterations to the peripheral metabolism of thyroid hormone, and raised circulating concentrations of cortisol and growth hormone, are best regarded as physiological adaptations to the state of starvation and do not require treatment. However, some medical complications are not only clinically important but are also life-threatening; these require special attention. Serious complications occur more commonly in the chronic patient who is emaciated, abuses laxatives, and induces vomiting. The total body vitamin and mineral deficiencies that can be so dangerous are often evident only when initial feeding unbalances the patient's precarious equilibrium.

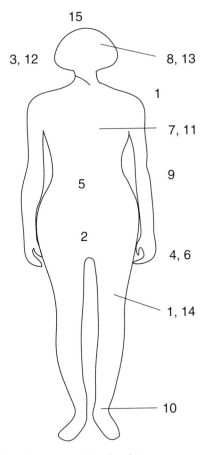

Figure 4.1. Physical signs of the eating disorders.

1. wAsting
2. laNugo hair
3. hypOthermia
4. Russell's sign
5. hypErcarotenemia
6. Xerosis
7. mItral valve prolapse
8. pArotid hypertrophy
9. lateNt tetany
10. dElayed relaxation of the tendon jerks
11. bRadycardia
12. Volume depletion
13. Organic brain syndrome
14. bruiSing
15. hAir loss

Table 4.1. *Medical complications of anorexia nervosa*

Metabolic

Hypothermia, dehydration

Electrolyte disturbances (hypokalemia, hypomagnesemia, hypocalcemia, hypophosphatemia)

Hypercholesterolemia

Hypoglycemia, raised liver enzymes

Cardiovascular

Hypotension, bradycardia, prolonged corrected QT interval, arrhythmia

Decreased myocardial wall thickness

Attenuated response to exercise

Pericardial effusion

Neurological

Pseudoatrophy of the brain

Abnormal electroencephalogram, seizures

Peripheral neuropathy

Compression neuropathy

Impaired autonomic function

Hematological

Anemia: usually normochromic normocytic

Leukopenia, thrombocytopenia

Iron-deficiency anemia

Megaloblastic anemia due to folate, vitamin B12, or rarely copper deficiency

Hypocellular bone marrow

Scurvy

Renal

Pre-renal azotemia

Partial diabetes insipidus

Acute and chronic renal failure

Endocrine

Low gonadotropins, estrogens, testosterone

Sick euthyroid syndrome

Raised cortisol, positive dexamethasone suppression test

Raised growth hormone

Musculoskeletal

Cramps, tetany, muscle weakness

Osteopenia, stress fractures

Gastroenterological

Swollen salivary glands, dental caries, erosion of enamel (with vomiting)

Superior mesenteric artery syndrome

Delayed gastric emptying, severe constipation, bowel obstruction

Irritable bowel syndrome, melanosis coli (from laxative misuse)

Immunological

Decreased interleukin-1 and tumor necrosis factor alpha, leading to more severe bacterial infections (staphylococcal lung abscess, tuberculosis)

4.1 Neurological

Central nervous system

Cerebrovascular accident due to embolus from mitral valve prolapse.

Organic brain syndrome due to protein-calorie malnutrition, drugs, deficiencies (magnesium, calcium, phosphorus, thiamine, vitamin B12), and vitamin A toxicity.

Pseudoatrophy of the brain due to fluid shifts.

Decreased level of consciousness (see section 5.5).

Seizures (see section 5.8).

Spinal cord

Vitamin B12 deficiency (subacute combined degeneration of the cord causing dorsal column and pyramidal tract dysfunction, and resulting in impaired joint position sense, vibration sense, and upper motor neuron weakness).

Muscle

Proximal myopathy due to magnesium, calcium, potassium, or phosphorus deficiency, or malnutrition.

Peripheral nervous system

Sensorimotor neuropathy caused by vitamin B12 or pyridoxine deficiency, protein-calorie malnutrition, or B vitamin excess.

Pressure neuropathy (foot drop, meralgia paresthetica).

Frequency of complications

Common: organic brain syndrome, proximal myopathy.

Uncommon: pseudoatrophy of the brain, neuropathies, seizures, decreased level of consciousness.

Rare: pressure neuropathies, cerebrovascular accidents.

Nursing implications

- Muscle weakness is common and usually due to malnutrition. However, it may be due to other deficiencies, which may be brought on by feeding, and therefore laboratory tests have to be repeated.

- The organic brain syndrome seen in low-body-weight AN will significantly impair the patient's ability to understand even simple concepts. Thus, significant psychotherapy may not be possible until nutrition is well under way.
- The pseudoatrophy of the brain is likely to be due to volume depletion. It will reverse when the fluid status of the patient normalizes.
- When the patient is very malnourished, and particularly if they are sedated, attention must be given to preventing pressure sores and pressure neuropathies. Pressure neuropathies are most likely to occur over the ulnar nerve at the elbow, the radial nerve behind the upper arm, and the lateral peroneal nerve over the neck of the fibula.

Patient information

- Muscle weakness is usually due to malnutrition. Gaining weight will reverse it. Occasionally, it is due to specific vitamin or mineral deficiencies. Blood tests are needed to diagnose these. They are treated by giving vitamins and minerals.
- At low body weight, the brain does not function properly. Memory and concentration are impaired. Depression will be worsened and response to antidepressant medications will not be complete at low body weight.

4.2 Dental

Eating disorders can cause erosion of the teeth, staining of the teeth, gum recession, gum friability and bleeding, and tooth loss. Decalcification of the lingual, palatal, and posterior occlusive surfaces of the teeth is referred to as perimyolysis and results from erosion by gastric acid during vomiting. Because amalgams are resistant to acid, they become much more obvious as enamel erosion progresses. Increased temperature sensitivity and increased incidence of caries have also been reported, but they have not been confirmed in all studies.

Prevention: recognize dental disease. Encourage the patient to see a dentist who is knowledgeable about eating disorders and with whom they can build a rapport. Knowledge of the dental effects of induced vomiting can be a major motivating factor for recovery.

After vomiting, the patient should not brush their teeth until the matrix of the teeth has restabilized (about half an hour). Initially, the mouth should be rinsed with water. The teeth should be brushed with bicarbonate-containing toothpaste.

Patients with AN do not get viral or bacterial infections more frequently than normal people. However, they have a poorer response to bacterial infections. They may not mount a febrile response to bacterial infection. Scurvy (vitamin C deficiency) can occur in AN. This causes swollen and bleeding gums. If there is significant mitral valve prolapse with regurgitation, then the patient should be given antibiotic prophylaxis before dental procedures.

Frequency of complications

Usual: mild erosion of the teeth.
Common: erosion of teeth and gum recession.
Uncommon: severe erosion of the teeth, gum recession, and staining of the teeth.
Rare: loss of teeth and dental abscess.

Nursing implications

Tooth and gum disease is common in AN, particularly with associated vomiting. Patients should be warned of this complication. If they do vomit, the mouth should be rinsed immediately, but tooth brushing should be delayed for half an hour, as brushing will remove unstable tooth matrix. The patient should seek regular dental assessment and treatment. If the patient is uncomfortable about telling the dentist that they vomit, then the patient should tell the dentist that they have been informed they have esophageal reflux.

Patient information

- Tooth and gum disease is caused by malnutrition, poor eating, bingeing, and especially vomiting. After vomiting, wait 30 minutes before brushing the teeth.
- Tooth and gum disease can be lessened by improving nutrition, discontinuing vomiting, and ensuring good dental hygiene, including rinsing the mouth after vomiting and having regular dental check-ups. If you are uncomfortable about telling the dentist that you have an eating disorder, then simply tell them that your doctor says you regurgitate food at night.
- If your doctor tells you that your heart has a leaky valve due to your weight loss, then ask whether you need to have antibiotics before dental and medical procedures. If so, you should warn your dentist beforehand, otherwise the procedure may have to be canceled at the last minute.

4.3 Skin

The cutaneous manifestations of AN depend on three factors: the nutritional and caloric content of the foods ingested and omitted, purging techniques, and illness duration (Table 4.2).

Both protein-calorie malnutrition and specific nutritional deficiencies are responsible for many of the cutaneous signs of AN. Unless indicated otherwise, feeding and nutritional supplementation are the specific treatments required.

Xerosis

Xerosis (dry skin) is observed in most undernourished patients. Xerosis is believed to develop secondary to a general deficiency of vitamins and trace elements and may be associated with the sick euthyroid syndrome commonly seen in AN. Xerosis is exacerbated by frequent washing, observed in AN especially when associated with obsessive-compulsive disorder. Xerosis can be ameliorated with moisturizing ointments and creams, but it will not resolve without nutrition.

Lanugo hair (hypertrichosis)

Lanugo hair is fine, pale hair that appears in the setting of severe protein-calorie malnutrition of AN. Interestingly, it does not appear when starvation is due to other causes. Lanugo hair is distributed primarily on the back, abdomen, and forearms; it presents as fine, downy, minimally pigmented soft hairs, although it is darker in dark-skinned people. It develops in conjunction with AN-associated weight loss and resolves with restoration of normal total body fat. The diagnosis of lanugo hair is established clinically. Histologically, lanugo hair is indistinguishable from normal hair.

Telogen effluvium

Telogen effluvium manifests as generalized shedding of normal telogen club hairs and is induced by physical or psychological stress. In this condition, some hair follicles are abruptly converted from anagen to telogen. The anagen–telogen ratio shifts, resulting in increased shedding. Hair loss develops two to four months after the period of stress, often during episodes of acute weight loss. Examination of the scalp is normal and without inflammation.

Table 4.2. *Skin conditions according to common anatomical location*

Location	Skin manifestation	Etiology	Comments
Hair	Trichotillomania	Patchy hair loss due to patient pulling out own hair Non-inflammatory, non-scarring	Occasionally present Treatment with clomipramine effective in the short term Hair should grow back once behavior stops
	Telogen effluvium	Generalized shedding of normal telogen club hairs induced by physical or psychological stress	Commonly present Hair should grow back once stress is resolved
	Pili torti	Hair-shaft abnormality in which individual hairs are twisted up to 360° on their own axes	Uncommon May be due to hypercarotenemia or hypothyroidism
Nails	Nail dystrophy	Abnormal nail formation in the setting of protein-calorie malnutrition and specific deficiencies, including ferritin, B12, folate, zinc, magnesium, calcium, and phosphorus	Occasionally present Normal nails likely to grow back slowly once nutritional deficiencies resolved
	Koilonychia	Spooning of the nails (concave centrally and reflected upwards laterally) due to iron deficiency May also be associated with pallor and/or glossitis	Occasionally present Serum ferritin measurement recommended Dietary cause must not be presumed; gastrointestinal symptoms, self-phlebotomy, and fecal occult blood measurement should be considered

(cont.)

Table 4.2. (cont.)

Location	Skin manifestation	Etiology	Comments
Perioral/oral	Angular stomatitis	Fissuring of the oral commisure usually associated with riboflavin and other vitamin deficiencies, although fungal infection and habitual tongue licking should be excluded	Occasionally present Treatment with multiple vitamin tablets is recommended
	Acrodermatitis enteropathica (also hands)	Pustules, scaling, and erosions seen on the face and hands due to zinc deficiency	Uncommon Supplementation with oral zinc is effective treatment Consider that zinc deficiency may occur in the setting of prolonged copper supplementation because copper competes with zinc for absorption
	Scurvy (also legs)	Gingival hypertrophy and easy bleeding, due to vitamin C deficiency Also see ecchymoses, perifollicular hemorrhages, follicular keratotic plugs, and impaired wound healing	Uncommon Associated with anemia, subperiosteal hemorrhages, deep hemorrhages, and dehiscence of old wounds Treat with vitamin C supplementation
Periorbital	Purpura	Small red spots (petechiae) around the eyes in mask-like distribution due to trauma and breakage of small blood vessels during forceful vomiting	Commonly present May be due to other exertions that elevate intrathoracic pressure, such as forceful coughing
	Subconjunctival hemorrhage	Red eye due to bleeding beneath the conjunctiva as a result of blood vessel damage due to forceful vomiting	Commonly present Other causes of red eye must be excluded

(cont.)

Table 4.2. (cont.)

Location	Skin manifestation	Etiology	Comments
Hands	Russell's sign	Small scars or callosities on back of hand and digits Result from repeated rubbing of the skin against the upper incisors when the hand is placed in the mouth to induce vomiting	Commonly present Although the scars are not reversible, they may decrease in size when the behavior is discontinued
	Pomphylyx (neurodermatitis)	Tiny, itchy, fluid-filled vesicles commonly on the lateral aspect of the digits Precipitated by severe stress associated with AN	Uncommon
	Hypercarotenemia	Yellowing of the skin due to carotene deposition, often noted on palms and soles Elevated serum carotene is due to slowed hepatic breakdown of carotene resulting from reduced basal metabolic rate Aggravated by increased consumption of carotene, found in carrots, squash, and spinach	Commonly present Should be distinguished from other causes of yellow skin, such as jaundice, by the absence of a scleral color change Restoration of normal nutritional status will hasten carotene metabolism and bring about resolution
	Acrocyanosis	Cool hands and feet with purple discoloration associated with delayed capillary refill Presents in the context of severe protein-calorie malnutrition	Occasionally present Should resolve with feeding

(cont.)

Table 4.2. (cont.)

Location	Skin manifestation	Etiology	Comments
	Acrodermatitis enteropathica (also perioral)	Pustules, scaling, and erosions seen on the face and hands due to zinc deficiency	Uncommon Supplementation with oral zinc is effective treatment Consider that zinc deficiency may occur in the setting of prolonged copper supplementation because copper competes with zinc for absorption
	Perniosis	Flat, red lesions located symmetrically on the ends of the fingers, nose, and ears Precipitated by exposure to cold	Uncommon Generally self-limited Avoid cold exposure, and protect the affected areas
Trunk/back	Lanugo hair	Fine downy hair due to severe protein-calorie malnutrition of AN Interestingly, does not appear when starvation is due to other causes	Common Resolves with restoration of normal total body fat
	Drug eruptions	Many various skin eruptions may be associated with medications Drugs used as a method of purging include laxatives, enemas, emetics, diuretics, herbal remedies, and other "diet pills"	Occasionally present High degree of suspicion of medication abuse is necessary

(cont.)

Table 4.2. (cont.)

Location	Skin manifestation	Etiology	Comments
	Pellagra (also legs, hands)	Hyperpigmented, scaly plaques in sun-exposed areas (hands, face, shins) "Casal's necklace" refers to a characteristic plaque located around the neck Due to deficiency in niacin (vitamin B3) or tryptophan	Rare Dermatitis precedes more severe manifestations, including diarrhea, dementia, and death Nutritional supplementation
	Prurigo pigmentosa	Itchy, red papules that evolve into irregular hyperpigmentation Affected areas include back, neck, and chest Cause is unknown	Rare Ketosis produced by AN may contribute to pathogenesis
	Xerosis (also legs/calves)	Dry skin due to deficiency of vitamins and trace elements May be associated with sick euthyroid syndrome	Commonly present Ameliorated with moisturizing ointments and creams, but will not resolve without restoration of normal nutritional status
Legs/calves	Scurvy (also oral and any location)	Bruising, perifollicular hemorrhages, and follicular keratotic plugs Also see impaired wound healing, gingival hypertrophy, and easy bleeding Scurvy is due to vitamin C deficiency	Uncommon Associated with anemia, subperiosteal hemorrhages, deep hemorrhages, and dehiscence of old wounds Treat with vitamin C supplementation
	Edema	Fluid retention often occurring during refeeding because of low basal metabolic rate	Commonly present Refeeding edema is due to fluid shifts and should not be treated aggressively

(cont.)

59

Table 4.2. (cont.)

Location	Skin manifestation	Etiology	Comments
		May also be due to intermittent fluid depletion associated with bingeing and purging, which causes the renin – angiotensin – aldosterone axis to be stimulated inappropriately	See previous section
	Xerosis (also trunk)	Dry skin due to deficiency of vitamins and trace elements	Commonly present
		May be associated with sick euthyroid syndrome	Ameliorated with moisturizing ointments and creams, but will not resolve without restoration of normal nutritional status
	Pellagra (also trunk, hands)	Hyperpigmented, scaly plaques in sun-exposed areas (hands, face, shins)	Rare
		Due to deficiency in niacin (vitamin B3) or tryptophan	Dermatitis precedes more severe manifestations, including diarrhea, dementia, and death
			Nutritional supplementation
Any location	Dermatitis artefacta	Bizarre-shaped lesions scattered irregularly over any body surface, due to self-inflicted harm (slashing, head hitting, or burning)	Commonly present
			Diagnosis of self-harm is difficult because patients are often reluctant to admit to the self-inflicted nature of the lesion
		Lesions may include excoriations, ulcers, bruising, round-shaped skin excavations, and scars	Careful history of depression and suicidal ideation must be obtained, and psychological treatment given

(cont.)

Table 4.2. (cont.)

Location	Skin manifestation	Etiology	Comments
	Self-phlebotomy	Needle track marks present over the veins from which blood has been drawn Antecubital fossa is the most common location	Occasionally present Measurement of serum hemoglobin (as frequent self-phlebotomy can lead to severe anemia) Treatment with loxapine may reduce behavior
	Erythema ab igne	Irregular hyperpigmented "lacy" area(s) on any surface area, resulting from the chronic application of hot water bottles or other heating devices by patient to warm themselves Constant feeling of cold associated with starvation-induced hypothermia	Occasionally present Hyperpigmentation is usually irreversible, despite behavior modification Malignant transformation within the patch has been reported
	Pruritus	Itchy skin and excoriations due to starvation-induced xerosis, dysfunction of cutaneous immunity, or enhanced levels of opioid activity	Occasionally present Rehydration of skin with ointments and creams and low-dose antihistamines
	Scurvy (also legs and oral)	Bruising, perifollicular hemorrhages, follicular keratotic plugs, impaired wound healing, gingival hypertrophy, and easy bleeding Scurvy is due to vitamin C deficiency	Uncommonly present Associated with anemia, subperiosteal hemorrhages, deep hemorrhages, and dehiscence of old wounds Treat with vitamin C supplementation

61

Pruritus

Starvation-associated pruritis is an important cutaneous sign in AN. Causes of AN-associated pruritus include xerosis, malnutrition-induced dysfunction of cutaneous immunity, and enhanced levels of opioid activity demonstrated in undernourished patients. Clinically, the patient may present with cutaneous lichenification and excoriations without an identifiable cutaneous abnormality. Therapeutic modalities include rehydration of the skin with ointments and creams and low-dose antihistamines.

Hypercarotenemia

Hypercarotenemia results from carotene deposition in the tissues, causing yellowing of the skin. Elevated serum carotene is due to a lowered basal metabolic rate in AN, with a resultant slowed hepatic breakdown of carotene. Hypercarotenemia is aggravated further by an increased consumption of carotene, found in some low-calorie foods, including carrots, squash, and spinach. Hypercarotenemia should be distinguished from other causes of yellow skin, such as jaundice. Pigmentation due to carotene can be differentiated from jaundice by palmar/plantar accentuation and the absence of a scleral color change (scleral icterus develops in jaundice because bilirubin has a high affinity for elastin-rich scleral tissue). Hypercarotenemia may also be observed in hypothyroidism and childhood, which are also associated with reduced hepatic metabolism. Hypercarotenemia is not seen in weight loss due to malabsorption, which is associated with low serum carotene levels. Patients should be reassured that hypercarotenemia does not have pathological consequences and that nutrition will hasten carotene metabolism and bring about resolution of this pigmentary disturbance.

Edema

Peripheral edema often occurs during feeding because the low metabolic rate associated with AN predisposes to fluid retention. Fluid retention can be significant, amounting to more than 10 kg. Excess fluid is most evident in dependent subcutaneous tissues, and is therefore most prominent in the feet of an ambulatory patient or over the sacrum of the bedridden patient. Refeeding edema is "pitting" edema and can be confirmed clinically by the persistence of an indentation following release of constant moderate pressure applied over a bony prominence in the edematous area. Pitting edema may also develop in BN, pregnancy, congestive heart failure, and hypoalbuminemia associated with renal protein wasting, a protein-losing enteropathy, or liver disease. Refeeding edema is due to fluid shifts and should not be treated aggressively. Diuretics should be avoided because they result in cyclically recurrent edema over a prolonged time period. Abstaining from excessive salt consumption and observing the patient for about two weeks is appropriate conservative management, allowing for the edema to resolve on its own.

Acrocyanosis

Acrocyanosis manifests clinically as violaceous, cool hands and feet and is associated with delayed capillary refill. Acrocyanosis presents in the context of severe protein-calorie malnutrition and is not associated with any histopathologic abnormalities.

Nail dystrophy

Abnormal nail formation is often seen in the setting of protein-calorie malnutrition and with many specific deficiencies, including ferritin, vitamin B12, folate, zinc, magnesium, calcium, and phosphorus. Nail dystrophy may be present in digits unequally, making it difficult to distinguish this from fungal infections of the nails.

Koilonychia

Koilonychia is "spooning of the nails," a deformity causing the nail to become concave centrally and reflected upwards laterally. Koilonychia is a consequence of iron deficiency and may be associated with pallor and a hypochromic microcytic anemia. Iron deficiency may also cause glossitis associated with flattening of the papillae of the tongue. Eating disorder patients often exclude red meat from their diet, and menstruation, if present, may contribute to loss of iron. Serum ferritin can be measured to confirm the diagnosis of iron deficiency. It is necessary to investigate carefully the cause of iron deficiency in all patients. A dietary cause must not be presumed, and a history of gastrointestinal symptoms, self-phlebotomy, and fecal occult blood measurement should be considered.

Angular stomatitis

Angular stomatitis, or perleche, is fissuring of the oral commisure. Although usually associated with riboflavin and other vitamin deficiencies, fungal infection and habitual tongue licking should be excluded. Laboratory measures of riboflavin are not widely available, and riboflavin deficiency is often part of multiple vitamin and mineral deficiencies; therefore, treatment with multiple vitamin tablets is recommended.

Acrodermatitis enteropathica

Acrodermatitis enteropathica is the name given to the cutaneous manifestations of zinc deficiency. It presents as periorificial and acral pustules, scaling, and erosions. There may also be associated changes in taste (dysgeusia), diffuse alopecia, and angular stomatitis. The pathology reveals acanthosis, parakeratosis, and ballooning degeneration of mid-epidermal keratinocytes. In the treatment of AN, it is important to consider that zinc deficiency may occur in the setting of prolonged copper supplementation, because copper competes with zinc for absorption. Supplementation with oral zinc is an effective treatment for zinc deficiency.

Pellagra

Pellagra presents as hyperpigmented and scaly plaques in a photodistribution over the hands, face, shins, and other sun-exposed areas. "Casal's necklace" refers to a characteristic, well-demarcated, hyperpigmented plaque located around the neck. Pellagra is due to a deficiency in either niacin (vitamin B3) or tryptophan. Niacin is a component of the electron transport chain and is essential for glycolysis and other metabolic processes. The dermatitis generally precedes more severe manifestations of pellagra, including diarrhea, dementia, and death. The histopathology of pellagra is indistinguishable from acrodermatitis enteropathica.

Scurvy

Scurvy results from vitamin C deficiency. Vitamin C is a cofactor necessary for the hydroxylation of proline and lysine in collagen biosynthesis. A deficiency of vitamin C has vascular, oral, and dermatological manifestations. Patients develop a tendency towards easy bleeding, and many develop ecchymoses, gingival hypertrophy, perifollicular hemorrhages, follicular keratotic plugs, and impaired wound healing. There may also be associated anemia, subperiosteal hemorrhages, deep hemorrhages, and dehiscence of old wounds. Outcome is fatal if not treated. Vitamin C blood levels are not widely available. Treat with 500–1000 mg of vitamin C daily for three weeks, and then give a multiple vitamin containing at least 10 mg of vitamin C daily.

Dermatologic features of the behavioral manifestations associated with anorexia nervosa

Recognition of the cutaneous features resulting from the behavioral manifestations of AN may facilitate an earlier diagnosis. Dermatologic manifestations associated with AN behavior include the following:

Erythema ab igne

Erythema ab igne manifests as an irregular, fixed, reticulated, hyperpigmented patch and is due to the chronic application of hot water bottles or other heating devices. Patients with AN often warm themselves because of a constant feeling of cold associated with starvation-induced hypothermia. This condition can be distinguished histopathologically from other dermatoses. Hyperpigmentation is usually irreversible, despite behavior modification. Rarely, malignant transformation within the patch has been reported.

Self-phlebotomy

The AN patient who self-phlebotomizes as a means of losing weight or causing self-harm will have needle track marks present over the veins from which blood has been drawn. The antecubital fossa is the most common location. Because frequent self-phlebotomy can lead to severe anemia, measurement of serum hemoglobin is recommended, and further treatment may be necessary. Most AN patients who practice self-phlebotomy are health care professionals. Treatment with loxapine is often effective in extinguishing this unusual practice.

Dermatitis artefacta

Self-inflicted harm may include slashing, head-hitting, or burning and may result in bizarre-shaped excoriations, ulcers, bruising, round-shaped skin excavations, and scars scattered irregularly over any body surface. Diagnosis of self-harm is often difficult because patients are reluctant to admit to the self-inflicted nature of their skin lesions. Ecchymoses may prompt a consideration of scurvy or coagulopathy, while healed cigarette burns on the legs may resemble diabetic dermatopathy. Many patients practice self-harm to dull their emotional pain with physical pain; therefore, once a diagnosis is established, psychological treatment should be given, and a careful history of depression and suicidal ideation must be obtained.

Trichotillomania

Patients with trichotillomania (compulsive hair-pulling) have a non-inflammatory, non-scarring alopecia. The histopathology of trichotillomania is distinct, demonstrating trichomalacia. Treatment with clomipramine is an effective short-term treatment.

Rare skin manifestations

Acne

One study of cutaneous findings in 14 patients with AN noted the onset of acne following feeding weight gain. The acne developed at a weight that, in these patients, was previously not associated with acne. The authors suggest a mechanism related to the re-establishment of physiological homeostasis.

Prurigo pigmentosa

Prurigo pigmentosa is a rare inflammatory disease of unknown etiology characterized by pruritic erythematous papules that evolve into a reticular hyperpigmentation. Affected areas include the back, neck, and chest. A case of prurigo pigmentosa has been reported in association with AN. The authors suggest that the ketosis produced by AN may contribute to the pathogenesis of prurigo pigmentosa.

Pili torti

Pili torti, a hair shaft abnormality that results in hair that is twisted up to 360 degrees on its own axis, was previously reported in 82% of AN patients. The authors of this report hypothesized that pili torti may be due to hypercarotenemia or hypothyroidism.

Perniosis

Perniosis presents as inflammatory, erythematous to violaceous macules and patches located bilaterally and symmetrically on the proximal phalanges, the acral areas, the nose, and the ears. It develops secondary to an abnormal vascular reaction and is precipitated by exposure to cold. Associations between AN and perniosis have been reported. It has been suggested that perniosis in AN is related to altered mechanisms of temperature control and vasoreactivity. Perniosis in AN is generally self-limited; treatment consists of avoiding cold exposure and protection of the affected areas.

Pomphylx

Pomphylx, also known as neurodermatitis, presents as pinpoint pruritic vesicles most prominently on the lateral aspect of the digits. Histologically, pomphylx is a spongiotic dermatitis with spongiotic vesicle formation. Neurodermatitis may be precipitated by severe stress associated with AN.

Eruptive neurofibromatosis

The rapid worsening of stable neurofibromatosis has been reported following the onset of AN in a single patient.

Signs associated with purging behavior

Russell's sign

Gerald Russell, in 1979, in his description of BN, noted the presence of callosities over the dorsum of the hand, resulting from repeated rubbing of the skin against the upper incisors. It is caused by the habitual induction of vomiting through the repeated placement of the hand in the mouth to induce emesis. There may be one to three scars distributed over the dorsal aspect of the digits as a result of repeated trauma induced by teeth as the digits of the dominant hand are forced down the throat. Russell's sign may also be seen in AN of the purging subtype. Histopathology demonstrates normal scar tissue. Although the scars are not reversible, they may decrease in size when induction of vomiting is discontinued.

Purpura

Forceful vomiting may cause trauma and breakage of the small vessels of the face, resulting in petechiae. Petechiae are often periocular and may have a mask-like distribution. Purpura may also be due to other exertions that elevate intrathoracic pressure.

Subconjunctival hemorrhage

Forceful vomiting can damage blood vessels in the eye and lead to subconjunctival hemorrhage.

Edema

The constant state of bingeing and purging can lead to intermittent fluid depletion, causing the renin–angiotensin–aldosterone axis to be stimulated inappropriately and leading to cyclic edema. This can be greatly disturbing to the patient, for the excess water will inevitably lead to a rapid rise in body weight, possibly increasing the drive to binge and purge. This edema will continue to recur until the binge–purge cycle is broken.

Drug eruptions

Patients with AN and BN may use various drugs as a method of purging. These medications include laxatives, enemas, emetics, diuretics, herbal remedies, and other "diet pills." Laxative abuse may lead to finger clubbing, thiazide diuretics may cause photosensitivity, ipecac has been implicated in a dermatomyolysis-like syndrome, and phenothiazines may cause a fixed drug eruption. Other possible drug-related dermatoses may also be seen, depending on the patient and drug characteristics. When taking the medical history, a high degree of suspicion of medication abuse is necessary.

Nursing implications

- Inspect skin for signs of self-harm and continue to search for and document any ongoing self-harm.
- Report any new rash to the physician.
- Use the treatment of any rash to build rapport. Patients are usually happy to receive advice and treatment of a rash.

Patient information

- Report any new rash to your physician.
- A rash may be a symptom of a deficiency state, the eating disorder, or self-harm behavior. All of these causes can be treated.

4.4 Respiratory

Lung function

The only significant changes are those of respiratory muscle weakness.

Pulmonary disorders

Aspiration pneumonia

Aspiration pneumonia is due to aspiration of the stomach contents. This is made more likely by a history of purging, a history of esophageal reflux, muscular weakness, a decreased level of consciousness, and a nasogastric tube in situ. The aspiration pneumonia may be chemical or bacterial. The chest radiograph is often normal for up to 24 hours after aspiration.

Bacterial pneumonia

Although viral and bacterial infections are no more likely in AN than in normal people, the response to bacterial infections is lessened in AN, such that there may be a reduced febrile response, making diagnosis more difficult. If dentition is poor, suspect an anaerobic cause. Progression to lung abscess and empyema is more likely than in normal people.

Other conditions

Spontaneous pneumothorax, pneumomediastinum, and subcutaneous emphysema can occur due to the repeated severe fluctuations in intrapulmonary pressure.

Frequency of occurrences

Uncommon: aspiration pneumonia, bacterial pneumonia that progresses to lung abscess or empyema, pulmonary muscle weakness, spontaneous pneumothorax, subcutaneous emphysema.

Rare: clubbing with no other cause apparent (causal association uncertain).

Nursing implications

- Respiratory complaints in AN are usually unrelated to AN itself and should be evaluated as in other patients.
- In the setting of tube feeding or a decreased level of consciousness, aspiration pneumonia may occur. Symptoms of cough, shortness of breath, and fever may be present. Because the febrile response to infection is less, and because AN patients tend to hypothermia in other situations, infection may be severe in the presence of an apparently normal body temperature. Therefore, a thorough medical assessment should be carried out. The chest X-ray may not show signs of aspiration pneumonia for 24 hours or more, and it is less likely to show changes if there is volume depletion.
- Cyanosis of the hands and feet is frequent with severe malnutrition with volume depletion. This is due to desaturation of blood due to the slow flow (stagnant hypoxia), and is not due to hypoxemia. Central cyanosis (involving the lips) is due to oxygen desaturation of hemoglobin. It should prompt a search for the usual causes of central cyanosis.

Patient information

- AN does not usually change lung function and has no long-term effects on the lungs.
- There is a small chance that regurgitation of nasogastric feedings given by a feeding tube might result in pneumonia.

• Blueness of the ends of the fingers and toes can be seen in AN and is corrected by treating dehydration and returning to a normal body weight.

4.5 Cardiovascular

About half of those patients with AN who die of the disease die suddenly, presumably of cardiac dysrhythmias. There have been only eight autopsies in AN reporting cardiac pathology, and there have been no prospective trials to determine which cardiac risk factors are more likely to cause death. However, we will summarize the information known, and give recommendations based primarily on experience.

Cardiac structure

Protein-calorie malnutrition causes decreased cardiac muscle mass and later myofibrillar degeneration of the endocardium and mitral valve prolapse. In addition, particularly if hypoalbuminemia coexists (although this is usually seen only when the quality of protein ingested is low), there may be a small pericardial effusion. These changes usually progress slowly with malnutrition and are therefore present in AN after months and are not present in BN (*vide infra*). All of these changes are reversible with weight gain.

Cardiac function

In the malnourished or bulimic patient, vitamin and mineral deficiencies can alter cardiac function. A vitamin B1 (thiamin) deficiency can cause wet beriberi with heart failure, although this is rare. Magnesium deficiency can cause dysrhythmia, prolongation of the QT interval, and congestive heart failure. Phosphate deficiency can cause rapid onset of congestive heart failure. During refeeding, serum phosphate levels can decrease rapidly, but phosphate deficiency is usually only of clinical significance once the serum level falls well below one-half the lower limit of normal. Deficiency of total body potassium predisposes to dysrhythmia and may worsen congestive heart failure. Very rarely, selenium deficiency will occur in long-term AN and can cause heart failure. Selenium deficiency occurs rarely, as the body has a large store of selenium. When it does occur, it is almost exclusively in people who eat produce grown from soil deficient in selenium (New Zealand, China, British Columbia, Canada). Anemia caused by folic acid, vitamin B12, iron, or copper deficiency will increase the work of the heart and worsen congestive heart failure in conjunction with another cause.

Protein-calorie malnutrition causes electrical changes, including abnormal cardiac pacing and changes in cardiac repolarization, resulting in prolongation of the QT interval, and ST and T wave abnormalities. The blood pressure is decreased, heart rate is low, and there may be changes in the autonomic function of the heart manifest by variability in heart rate and cardiac depolarization.

Of greatest concern in AN are cardiac dysrhythmias due to refeeding. It is during refeeding that the patient rapidly uses the limited stores of vitamins and minerals that they do have and frequently has falling levels of potassium, magnesium, and phosphate due to this rapid use.

Atherosclerosis

Patients with AN are amenorrheic, have high low-density lipoprotein (LDL) and low high-density lipoprotein (HDL) lipids and apoprotein abnormalities, frequently smoke, and are under a great deal of stress. All of these are predisposing factors to atherosclerosis in females. Three of the eight autopsies performed on anorexics showed significant atherosclerotic lesions. Patients with AN frequently have chest pain, often of more than one type. The causes of chest pain in AN include chest-wall pain, reflux esophagitis, esophageal spasm, chest pain due to abdominal bloating, and typical and atypical angina. Palpitations may be perceived as a chest pain. About 20% of patients interviewed in one study were found to have pain consistent with typical or atypical angina.

Medications

Drugs taken in prescribed psychopharmacotherapy or for self-harm include tricyclic antidepressants, major tranquilizers, prokinetic agents, erythromycin, and antihistamines. All of these can prolong the QT interval of the EKG and predispose to dysrhythmias and Torsade de pointes.

Bacterial endocarditis

Endocarditis is somewhat more likely in AN due to mitral valve prolapse, which may be associated with regurgitation and the characteristic mid-systolic murmur, dental caries, and polymorphonuclear leukocytic dysfunction related to magnesium deficiency, zinc deficiency, and severe protein-calorie malnutrition. However, this is rare.

Overdose and the heart

Overdose in AN has the same type of risk as in non-anorexic patients, except that the likelihood of dysrhythmias or heart failure is proportionally greater. Careful history of medications taken, including over-the-counter medications (e.g. antihistamines for sleep) should be taken.

Diagnosis

Hypotension

Blood pressure should be measured in AN and is commonly low – in the range of 90/70 mm Hg. This does not cause symptoms unless it is associated with volume depletion. If the jugular venous pressure is low, then this indicates volume depletion. Postural hypotension can occur without volume depletion due to impaired vascular and autonomic responsiveness. Hypothermia, which commonly occurs in AN, can also cause hypotension and lack of vascular responsiveness.

Variability in heart rate

Heart rate is usually low in AN – in the range of 45–60 per minute. However, particularly if the patient is an athlete, the heart rate may be as low as 30 per minute. As long as there are no symptoms, this does not increase morbidity or mortality. Variable heart rate or changes in conduction may indicate autonomic dysfunction and may be an indicator of an increased likelihood of sudden death. Heart sounds are normal in AN. They sound somewhat loud due to the thin chest wall. Mitral valve prolapse, which occurs in about 17% of healthy young women, is even more common in AN; it worsens as malnutrition worsens, and it improves as malnutrition improves. Therefore, the mid-systolic clicks may increase in number and be associated with a murmur, and eventually there may be significant regurgitation due to mitral valve prolapse. This is reversible with feeding. Mitral valve prolapse is best heard with the patient standing and doing the Valsalva maneuver.

Electrocardiographic abnormalities

Most patients with AN have a normal EKG, apart from bradycardia, but first-degree heart block, ectopic atrial rhythms, nodal escape, ventricular premature complexes, ST depression, and U waves may all occur. Most of these abnormalities will normalize within two weeks of correcting deficiencies and feeding. No other treatment for cardiac abnormalities has been subjected to a clinical trial. Our anecdotal experience is that none should be used except for dysrhythmias that meet the usual cardiological criteria for clinical importance. In this case, we recommend cardiac monitoring until the abnormality resolves (usually within 72 hours) and giving metoprolol 25–100 mg. The QTc interval (the QT interval corrected for heart rate) is usually prolonged with weight loss. It will commonly be in the range of 350–400 ms in young females. Patients with AN and who die of dysrhythmias may have QTc intervals in this range. In our opinion, the relative prolongation of the QTc interval that occurs with weight loss, mineral deficiencies, or drugs is a predisposing factor to dysrhythmias. Therefore, the QTc interval need not be 550 ms, the length usually of concern in adults, to be significant. Until further evidence is available, we recommend caution if the QTc is more than 450 ms or 60 ms longer than at baseline. Comparison with a baseline EKG is important. Also, changes in T waves, pacemaker function, rhythmicity, and other changes may occur so that the EKG may appear bizarre. In the absence of symptoms, volume or mineral deficiencies, or medications, this is likely to be due to malnutrition alone. If these other situations pertain, then the changes may be related to medications or mineral deficiencies. Presentation with collapse should be considered to be due to a dysrhythmia until proved otherwise.

Differential diagnosis

Valvular dysfunction due to the use of anorectic medications should be considered if there is a history of taking D-fenfluramine or L-fenfluramine and phentermine for more than three months. An echocardiogram should be done to exclude valvular dysfunction in this setting. Hyperthyroidism, which can worsen the symptoms of eating disorder, can also predispose to dysrhythmia. In the differential diagnosis of AN, Addison's disease, which may cause hyperkalemia and hyponatremia, should be considered. There is some evidence that repeated doses of ipecac may cause a cardiomyopathy, although this is uncertain. In any case, a history of ipecac use should be taken.

Nursing implications

- Cardiac arrhythmia is the most common medical cause of death from AN.
- Heart function is usually normal in AN. However, the heart wall is usually thinned and the mitral valve usually has an increased (although insignificant) leak (clicks or murmur).
- The electrical recovery of the conduction system of the heart is measured by the QTc interval, which is reported on the EKG printout. In AN, the QTc is often prolonged, which increases the chance of arrhythmia and sudden death. Report to the physician a QTc greater than 450 ms.

- Heart failure can occur if the serum phosphorus drops to less than one-half the lower limit of normal. Contact the physician if the serum phosphorus drops below normal.
- Monitor heart rate and blood pressure lying down and then sitting or standing, because the effect of medications, dehydration, and AN may not be evident when lying down.
- Variability of heart rate that is not caused by standing, exercise, or anxiety may be due to dysfunction of the autonomic nervous system, which increases the chance of arrhythmias.

Patient information

- Report chest pain, palpitations, and dizziness to your nurse or doctor, because these may be symptoms of heart involvement from the eating disorder.
- The cardiac complications of AN are reversible.

4.6 Gastrointestinal

Salivary glands

Parotid and submandibular gland enlargement is a classic finding in both AN and BN, and may be the only due to diagnosis on physical examination. It may occur with protein-calorie malnutrition itself, but it is more likely to occur and is more marked with vomiting. Purging may cause salivary gland hypertrophy by increased pressure of salivary fluid building up behind the swollen papillae where fluid empties into the mouth. Resolution of parotid and salivary gland hypertrophy after successful treatment of the eating disorder is the norm, although this can take several months. Using warming over the parotid gland and irrigating the mouth with saline and lemon may hasten normalization. Rarely, unilateral tender swelling of a parotid gland will occur. Acute suppurative parotitis due to infection of the parotid gland with *Staphylococcus aureus* should be considered. This occurs rarely if adequate hydration and good mouth hygiene are maintained.

Hyperamylasemia, due to release of the enzyme amylase from the salivary glands, occurs after purging. Serum amylase also comes from the pancreas, the urogenital epithelium, and the small bowel mucosa. Therefore, lipase, which comes only from the pancreas, should be measured in eating disorder patients to exclude pancreatitis, if this is being considered. Alternatively, the tissue of origin of the increased amylase can be determined by measuring amylase isoenzymes.

Esophagus

Abnormal peristalsis, decreased lower esophageal sphincter tone, free reflux, esophagitis, and even esophageal rupture (Boerhave's syndrome) can occur with vomiting. Boerhave's syndrome is a catastrophic manifestation requiring emergency medical and surgical intervention. Chronic sequelae of recurrent vomiting include the development of esophageal strictures or Barrett's esophagus. Barrett's esophagus is the replacement of the normal epithelium of the esophagus with squamous epithelium. This precancerous state requires endoscopic follow-up. Mallory–Weiss tears may lead to significant gastrointestinal bleeding. These tears at the junction between the stomach and the esophagus are caused by the physical trauma of vomiting. Lesser degrees of esophageal dysfunction are seen with malnutrition alone. If bisphosphonates are used to treat osteoporosis, then care must be taken to avoid the possible associated esophagitis and esophageal stricture.

Stomach

Decreased and impaired motility are frequent. This can result in gastric stasis, early satiety, and a predisposition to esophageal reflux. Acute gastric dilation and rupture have been described in bulimics during bingeing and in anorexics during refeeding. Rapid onset of nausea, vomiting, or abdominal pain may indicate gastric distension; in most cases, this can be treated conservatively by nasogastric suction and fluid and electrolyte replacement. In extreme cases, gastric rupture can occur, causing dramatic pain, sepsis, and shock, and requiring urgent surgical intervention.

Small and large bowel

AN and other eating disorder patients often have slow and abnormal peristalsis. This can result in postprandial bloating, increased intestinal gas, constipation, fecal impaction, and paradoxical diarrhea (overflow diarrhea). Laxative abuse can cause or exacerbate symptoms, since chronic use of stimulant laxatives may result in loss of normal peristaltic function. Laxative abusers usually complain of periods of diarrhea alternating with episodes of constipation. Cathartic colon can become severe and may even necessitate colonic resection. Chronic, recurrent use of laxatives may result in gastrointestinal bleeding, ranging from occult to frank blood loss. Celiac disease and inflammatory bowel disease may coexist with AN but are not made more likely by its presence. Rectal prolapse, fecal impaction, and fecal incontinence can occur in chronic AN due to weakness of the muscles of the pelvic floor.

Liver and gallbladder

These organs are usually normal. A fatty liver can occur with severe protein malnutrition. Gallbladder contraction may be slow. Production of cholesterol-containing gallstones is more likely with recurrent weight loss.

Pancreas

The pancreas is usually normal. There is no need for pancreatic enzyme tests. Type I diabetes mellitus may coexist with AN. Acute pancreatitis can develop in BN and in the purging form of AN. Alcohol ingestion and biliary tract disease, both of which may complicate eating disorders, are the most likely reasons for this association. If signs or symptoms of pancreatitis, such as abdominal pain, nausea, or vomiting are observed, then measurement of serum amylase and isoenzymes will suggest the correct diagnosis. The abdominal pain may go unnoticed because of a history of abdominal complaints, and the amylase may be elevated due to purging. Therefore, serum lipase should be measured and an ultrasound of the pancreas ordered to confirm the diagnosis. When pancreatitis is diagnosed, treatment with bowel rest, nasogastric suction, and intravenous fluid replacement should be instituted promptly.

Digestion

Digestion is normal unless the patient is using laxatives, in which case rapid transit of food may cause about a 4% reduction in the absorption of calories.

Frequency of occurrences

Usual: decreased gastric and intestinal motility with postprandial bloating, constipation, salivary gland enlargement involving both the parotid and submandibular glands.
Common: paradoxical diarrhea.
Uncommon: esophagitis.
Rare: peptic ulcer, esophageal stricture, Barrett's esophagus, Boerhaave's syndrome, esophageal rupture, fatty liver, rectal prolapse.

Nursing implications

• Abdominal bloating, gas, and excessive fullness after eating are almost always seen and will improve with regular eating, adequate but not excessive fluid intake, and prokinetic agents if required.

- There is no change in the patient's ability to absorb foods or the ability of their liver or pancreas to function in digestion. They do not need bile or pancreatic supplements.
- Patients who have a history of laxative abuse may have very little intestinal peristalsis. They will require special attention, including the laxative withdrawal protocol.

Patient information

- You can expect to have some bloating and cramps and irregularity of bowel movements because your bowel is weakened. However, this will improve as your weight and eating habits improve.
- You may require medication to help your bowel return to normal. Your physician may prescribe this. If you use only the medications prescribed to you, your bowels will recover faster.
- AN does not cause any permanent damage to your bowel or digestive system, but the persistent use of purgatives may do so.

4.7 Endocrine

Hypothalamic/pituitary

Hypothalamic/pituitary changes are secondary to weight loss. Follicle-stimulating hormone (FSH) and luteinizing hormone (LH) may drop to prepubertal levels, resulting in amenorrhea in females. There may be some reduction in antidiuretic hormone, resulting in partial diabetes insipidus. All of these changes reverse with feeding, and so they should not be treated. Dopamine antagonists cause an increase in prolactin, which may cause decreased libido, breast engorgement, and lactation.

Thyroid

The metabolic rate is adjusted downward (sick euthyroid syndrome) as a consequence of low levels of the active thyroid hormones (T4 and T3), an increase in inactive thyroid hormone (reverse tri-iodothyronine, rT3), and a level of TSH that is within normal range. This is a physiological adaptation to malnutrition; it is not hypothyroidism and should not be treated. Rarely, hyperthyroidism will occur at the same time as AN. If it does, it will exacerbate the symptoms of AN and may be occult because its symptoms are similar to those of AN.

Adrenal

The hypothalamic-pituitary-adrenal axis has been evaluated less extensively in patients with BN than in patients with AN. Most studies have found that plasma cortisol and ACTH levels in bulimics are similar to those of controls. Others have reported that a subset of bulimic women with normal weight have elevated plasma cortisol and ACTH levels with blunted responses to corticotrophin releasing factor (CRF). Non-suppression on the dexamethasone test occurs in some bulimic patients.

Ovarian

Amenorrhea occurs, but is secondary to hypothalamic/pituitary dysfunction and decreased conversion of hormones by the fat mass, leading to low circulating levels of pituitary gonadotropins. Even with amenorrhea, ovulation may still take place. Pregnancy must therefore still be protected against. Because the menstrual disturbance often precedes severe weight loss and may persist after weight is regained, other factors must also be involved. These include a disturbance of estrogen metabolism and a fault in estrogen feedback to the hypothalamus.

The demonstration by pelvic ultrasound of a resumption of the formation of ovarian follicles presages the return of normal endocrine function, which occurs in patients who regain and maintain a normal weight. Pelvic ultrasound can thereby be used to help determine whether a physiologically normal weight has been attained in the absence of menses. However, the likelihood of a normal pregnancy is poor in patients who conceive before they have recovered fully from their illness. Low birth weight and a higher incidence of spontaneous abortion, congenital malformations, prematurity, and perinatal mortality, together with poor parenting, have been reported. Induction of pregnancy by methods such as pulsatile luteinizing hormone-releasing hormone (LHRH) is thus injudicious. Reproductive function after recovery, however, is usually normal.

Menstrual abnormalities are also seen in normal-weight patients with BN, although less frequently than in AN. In BN, a pattern of irregular menses is more common than amenorrhea. A decreased number of LH secretory spikes and abnormal LH responses to gonadotropin-releasing hormones have been reported in some bulimic patients.

Genital

Breast size regresses in adults and does not progress in prepubertal females. If medications are used that cause an increase in prolactin, then breast engorgement and lactation may occur.

Temperature regulation

Hypothermia is common, as is a decreased response to pyrogens.

Leptin

Leptin levels are reduced, but only in proportion to adipose tissue mass.

Gut hormones

Gut hormones are normal.

Peroxisome proliferator-activated receptor

Peroxisome proliferator-activated receptor (PPAR) is normal.

Pancreatic endocrine hormone production

Pancreatic endocrine hormone production is normal.

Hypoglycemia

Hypoglycemia is particularly troublesome during refeeding. In healthy subjects, ingestion of a meal containing glucose results in a rise in serum glucose followed by pancreatic secretion of insulin to move glucose into cells. To prevent the blood glucose level from dropping too low, glucagon is secreted from the pancreas, causing the liver to release glucose from its stores of glycogen. In AN, the glycogen stores in the liver are depleted. As a result, when refeeding begins and insulin is secreted, hypoglycemia may result. This low blood sugar, or hypoglycemia, can cause headaches, confusion, impaired level of consciousness, seizures, and death. If these symptoms occur during refeeding, then the blood sugar should be measured between meals and at night. A blood glucose level of less than 2.5 mmol/l is diagnostic of hypoglycemia. Alternatively, a glucagon test can be performed. In the fasting state, blood glucose is measured before, and ten and 20 minutes after, intravenous administration of 1mg of glucagon. A normal response is an elevation of glucose above 7 mmol/l. Hypoglycemia is treated with refeeding an intravenous dextrose to maintain the blood sugar above 5 mmol/l. Thiamine must be administered intravenously and orally in a dose of 100 mg each followed by 100 mg orally for ten days. Thiamine must be given to avoid precipitating Wernicke's encephalopathy with the dextrose infusion.

Frequency of occurrences

Usual: amenorrhea, infertility, hypothermia, reduction in breast tissue, reduction in libido, hypoglycemia.

Common: ovulation and therefore fertility present with amenorrhea, sick euthyroid syndrome, hyperprolactinemia due to medications.

Rare: partial diabetes insipidus, exacerbation of AN by concurrent hyperthyroidism of any cause.

Nursing implications

- Loss of menstruation in a female patient does not mean that she is not ovulating. She may still be ovulating and thus may get pregnant. She must take steps at birth control.
- It is uncertain whether use of the oral contraceptive pill will help to reduce osteoporosis in AN.
- Decreasing breast size in postpubertal female patients is normal. This will reverse with weight recovery.
- In the prepubertal female with AN, breast development will be halted.

Patient information

- If having no periods is bothersome to you, your doctor can prescribe the oral contraceptive pill.
- Even though you are not menstruating, you may still be ovulating and could get pregnant. You must use birth control.
- A decrease in breast size (or, if you have not gone through puberty yet, a halt in breast development) is normal in AN. With recovery, breast development will resume.

4.8 Renal

Renal function

Reduced fluid intake and reduced concentrating ability of the kidney may result in increased urinary frequency and nocturia, decreased urine volume, and predisposition to renal stones (also because of increased urinary ketones due to adipose tissue breakdown). The urinary concentrating ability can be reduced by concurrent psychogenic polydipsia. Due to the marked reduction in lean body mass, the serum creatinine is lower than normal. However, the creatinine clearance will reflect the normal renal function. Renal insufficiency occasionally develops as a consequence of vomiting and laxative misuse, with associated electrolyte disturbances.

Prolonged purging and/or diuretic or laxative abuse can result in a hypo-volemic state that stimulates the renin–angiotensin–aldosterone system, as homeostatic mechanisms attempt to conserve fluids. When the patient attempts to curtail diuretic or laxative use, persistent hyperaldosteronism results in edema formation. Unfortunately, this often triggers severe anxiety about weight gain and resumption of diuretic or laxative abuse. This self-perpetuating cycle can be extremely difficult to interrupt, and the patient must be reassured that fluid retention is a temporary condition that will resolve if purging behaviors can be avoided. Dependent edema should be treated by reassurance; it will disappear without treatment in a week or two. Bedrest and below-knee anti-embolic stockings may be used. If significant fluid retention (e.g. more than 10 kg) threatens compliance, then drug therapy may be necessary. Spironolactone, which is a weak physiologic aldosterone antagonist, can be given in doses of between 50 and 200 mg a day to be tapered over two weeks. Alternatively, an angiotensin-converting enzyme inhibitor may be employed. However, the risk of hyperkalemia and renal insufficiency limit its usefulness in AN.

With severe AN, the muscles of the pelvis will be weak and a mild degree of neuropathic bladder may occur due to a neuropathy (see Section 4.1). This predisposes to urinary retention, stress incontinence, and lower urinary tract infections.

Frequency of complications

Usual: nocturia, frequency.
Common: mild azotemia (usually only due to volume depletion).
Uncommon: psychogenic polydipsia, urinary incontinence.
Rare: renal stones, neuropathic bladder.

Nursing implications

Nocturia is common and is related to malnutrition and decreased urinary concentrating ability. It disappears with feeding.

Patient information

- Passing urine at night is common in AN. It is due to a reduction in the ability of your kidney to concentrate urine. This disappears with weight recovery.
- It is important to drink enough fluid, but do not too much as this will adversely affect the levels of salts in your blood. Discuss with your doctor or dietician the volume of fluid you should be drinking.

4.9 Bones and joints

Bone

Decreased bone mass (osteoporosis and its precursor osteopenia) occurs in AN and worsens in relation to the degree of malnutrition and the length of disease. Dietary deficiency, low circulating estrogens, hypercortisolism, laxative misuse, and disturbed acid–base balance are thought to be responsible. Neither estrogen nor progesterone is useful in the treatment of osteopenia in AN. If AN occurs before full linear growth is completed and recovery does not occur before the epiphyses close, then height is reduced. With increasing osteoporosis, the risk of fracture is increased. Initially, stress fractures occur in weight-bearing bones in the feet, lower limbs, and pelvis. Later, vertebral fractures occur, with a reduction in body height and often chronic back pain. If osteomalacia occurs (reduced bone mineral mass), then a cause other than AN must be sought: AN by itself does not cause osteomalacia. Rarely, deficiency states due to AN will cause osteomalacia.

Joints

There are no abnormalities of the joints other than those that can result from overexercise.

Frequency of occurrences

Usual: decreased linear growth in adolescents, reduced bone mass.
Common: osteoporosis, stress fractures.
Uncommon: pelvic fractures, vertebral fractures.
Rare: osteomalacia (usually not caused by the AN).

Nursing implications

Osteoporosis is common is AN. Adequate intake of vitamin D and calcium must be encouraged, but only restoration of normal nutritional status has been shown to return bone mass to within normal limits.

Patient information

- AN causes weaker bones (osteoporosis). However, studies have shown that if patients return to normal weight, then bones can return to a normal strength.

- Bones continue building within themselves all your life. The lengthening of bones stops after the teen years.
- It is important to take vitamin D, calcium, and other medications as prescribed, but there is no substitute for weight recovery.

4.10 Hematological

Hemoglobin

Hemoglobin is usually slightly low due to the anemia of chronic disease. This is a secondary sideroblastic anemia that results from impaired transfer of iron to red blood cells in states of illness. The anemia may be due to a reduction in circulating stem cells. Anemia can also be due to deficiencies of iron, vitamin B12, folic acid, and rarely copper. Severe anemia can be caused by self-phlebotomy. Self-phlebotomy should be suspected if the level of hemoglobin drops quickly, if there is an associated iron deficiency but no associated deficiency in the diet, and also in the presence of unexplained needle marks. Almost all cases of self-phlebotomy occur in health care workers. Rarely, marrow failure will result from drug toxicity or even malnutrition. This can be life-threatening.

White blood cells

These are often moderately low secondary to protein-calorie malnutrition. The neutrophil count is well above the critical value for protection against bacterial infections (500 cells per mm^3). With deficiencies of vitamin B12, folate, or copper, a megaloblastic anemia occurs that causes large, multilobed polymorphonuclear leukocytes. Rarely, bone marrow failure occurs. In AN, this is usually associated with a more prominent decrease in hemoglobin than in white cells or platelets.

The lymphocyte count is normal. If the eosinophil count is increased (more than 500 cells per mm^3), suspect Addison's disease.

Platelets

Platelet count is usually normal. Platelets may be reduced in vitamin B12, folate, or copper deficiency, toxicity from drugs or alcohol, or bone marrow failure.

Vitamin K

Coagulopathies and trauma must be excluded as causes for bleeding. Vitamin K deficiency as a cause of coagulopathy in AN has not been reported. Vitamin K is a fat-soluble vitamin formed by bacterial flora. The vitamin K-dependent coagulation factors (II, VII, IX, X) are formed in the liver. Both of these mechanisms are relatively unaffected by AN.

Frequency of occurrences

Usual: mild anemia, leukopenia.
Common: iron-deficiency anemia.
Uncommon: anemia or leukopenia due to vitamin B12 or folate deficiency.
Rare: anemia from copper deficiency, anemia from self-phlebotomy, bone marrow failure due to drug toxicity.

Nursing implications

- Mild anemia and leukopenia are common in AN and usually require no special treatment other than refeeding.
- Mild leukopenia is not associated with an increased risk of infection.
- Deficiency states may result in severe anemia, low white cells, and low platelets, and may require specific treatment.

Patient information

A slight lowering of hemoglobin or white blood cells is common in AN. Usually, there are no ill effects. Unless due to deficiencies in vitamins or minerals or another disease, no treatment other than refeeding is required. Iron-deficiency anemia is common, especially if the diet is strictly vegetarian or vegan.

4.11 Immune

AN is not associated with any increased likelihood of contracting viral or bacterial infections. However, in AN the ability to respond to and recover from bacterial infections is reduced. The cause of this is not clear, although it may be related to reduced cellular mobility resulting from impaired cytokine production. There is a reduced febrile response to bacterial infection in AN.

Cellular

Impairment of cell-mediated immunity is seen only with very severe malnutrition. Magnesium deficiency causes white blood cells to be dysfunctional.

Zinc deficiency may cause decreased cellular function. Vitamin B12 and folate deficiencies can cause low white cells counts, rarely to a level (less than 500 cells per mm^3) where infection is more likely.

Antibody

Antibody production and amounts are normal.

Frequency of occurrences

Usual: slightly low neutrophil count of no significance.

Common: if bacterial infections occur, they are more virulent and are more likely to develop complications. This is particularly the case with bacterial pneumonia, which tends to progress to lung abscess and empyema more frequently in AN.

Uncommon: decreased cellular response due to magnesium or zinc deficiency.

Rare: agranulocytosis associated with bone marrow failure.

Nursing implications

- Immunity is normal in AN. Viral and bacterial infections do not occur more frequently. However, bacterial infections tend to be more severe.
- There is a decreased febrile response to infection in AN.

Patient information

- The immune system is normal in AN. You can receive vaccination as usual, and you are no more likely than other people to get a viral or bacterial infection.
- If you do get a bacterial infection (such as pneumonia or urinary tract infection), you may not have a fever and the infection may be more severe. You must therefore get treatment early for bacterial infections.

Chapter 5

The clinician's response to common physical complaints

Many of the physical symptoms of AN are related directly to the effects of semi-starvation, while other physical symptoms are associated mainly with behavioral problems such as excessive exercising, vomiting, and purging. Table 5.1 lists the most common physical manifestations in AN. Table 5.2 lists the physical manifestations most commonly found in BN.

5.1 Edema

Case

A 25-year-old female gains 10 kg in seven days. She is extremely anxious and agitated and threatens to discharge herself against medical advice. The nurse asks you why she has gained so much weight.

Comment

During feeding, edema occurs due to volume depletion, low metabolic rate, behaviors such as vomiting and laxative, enema, and diuretic use, which cause the body to have high circulating hormones that promote the retention of fluid. Antidiuretic hormone is secreted by the pituitary, renin is secreted by the kidney, angiotension is formed in the blood, and aldosterone is produced by the adrenal gland. The amount of fluid that might be retained in a patient is impossible to predict, but it is often 3–5 kg of water. The fluid retention is much greater in patients with a history of binge–purge behavior or diuretic use.

If the patient is suspected of having edema, apply steady, firm pressure with the pad of your thumb over the skin covering the lower tibia, just about the

Table 5.1. *Common physical symptoms of anorexia nervosa*

Gastrointestinal and urological
    Abdominal pain, constipation, heartburn, feelings of abdominal bloating,
      early satiety
    Frequent urination, nocturia
    Amenorrhea

Ear, nose, and throat
    Mouth pain due to dental cavities and gum disease
    Easy bleeding of gums
    Salivary gland hypertrophy

Dermatological
    Hair loss from scalp
    Fine hair growth on body
    Dry skin

Musculoskeletal
    Lack of growth
    Muscle weakness and cramping
    Bone pain

Central and autonomic nervous systems
    Fatigue, dizziness
    Hyperactivity
    Impaired concentration and short-term memory

Cardiovascular
    Slow heart and pulse rate
    Palpitations

General
    Tiredness
    Coldness, intolerance to cold environment
    Dizziness on standing
    Marked variation in weight with recurrent fluid retention
    Hypothermia, sensitivity to cold and heat due to diminished fat

---

ankle. After 15 seconds, a small pit will appear if edema is present. The depth of the pit is roughly proportional to the amount of edema if the patient has been ambulatory for hours. If the patient has been lying down, then the edema will shift to the most dependent area; this is usually the lower back. In this case, apply pressure in the midline over the lumbosacral spine.

Less commonly, edema is due to hypoalbuminemia (low oncotic pressure), renal failure (high creatinine with associated fluid retention), or heart failure.

Table 5.2. *Major physical symptoms of bulimia nervosa*

Gastrointestinal and urological
Abdominal pain, constipation
Heartburn, feelings of abdominal bloating, early satiety
Irregular menses
Dental
Dental decay
Dermatological
Russell's sign
Musculoskeletal
Usually none
Central and autonomic nervous systems
Fatigue, dizziness
Cardiovascular
Usually none
General
Tiredness
Dizziness on standing
Marked variation in weight with recurrent fluid retention

Prevention

Normalize the fluid volume on admission. If an intravenous line is not available, then salt-containing cubes dissolved in water can be ingested. As soon as the jugular venous pressure is normalized, discontinue the salt administration. Rest should be encouraged because recumbency allows the body to clear excess fluid by increasing the glomerular filtration rate. If the risk of edema is considered high or treatment resistance is felt to be very likely if edema occurs, give spironolactone 200 mg once a day for 14–21 days. Spironolactone is a weak diuretic that is a physiologic aldosterone antagonist. It interrupts the cause of the edema in most cases, and causes potassium and magnesium retention rather than the increased loss induced by most diuretics.

Treatment

If edema develops, reassure the patient that it is temporary and encourage bedrest. Treatment with diuretics often causes cyclic edema (continued recurrent edema), which may last for up to a year after discontinuing diuretics. If treatment is to be given, treat with spironolactone as above. If the edema is refractory to spironolactone, then second-line treatment is an angiotensin-converting enzyme inhibitor, such as enalapril. These medications decrease angiotension formation and thereby aldosterone production.

- Examine for edema: press softly with your thumb over a bony prominence of a dependent area to test for pitting edema.
- Consider feeding, hypoalbuminemia, congestive heart failure, and renal failure.
- Give information and reassurance.
- Encourage bedrest.
- If the edema leads to treatment resistance or refusal:

  - give spironolactone 200 mg a day for two to four weeks;
  - do not give other diuretics, as they will cause recurrent edema and thereby diuretic dependency.

Nursing implications

- Reassure the patient that edema is common and that it usually resolves in one to two weeks with no treatment.
- Have the patient rest in bed. This reduces the edema by increasing the fluid return to the blood and removal by the kidney.
- If spironolactone is used, tell the patient that it is a diuretic that blocks the cause of the edema. They will not need it more than two to four weeks.

5.2 Aches and pains

Case

A 28-year-old female with chronic AN is seen for aches and pains. She has been stable for several years. A few months ago, she began eating more in an attempt to improve her strength. She began having aches and pains about a month ago. She comes to see you to ask whether you can help.

Comment

"Aches and pains" can mean different things. It may mean weakness, muscle cramps, numbness, causalgic (burning) pain, bone pains, or non-specific systemic symptoms. Therefore, first define the problem. See Table 5.3 for the differential diagnosis.

Table 5.3. *Causes of aches and pains in patients with eating disorders*

Problem	Syndrome	Causes	Investigations	Treatment
Weakness	Proximal myopathy	Potassium deficiency Phosphorus deficiency Magnesium deficiency	Measure serum levels, may need to do magnesium load test	Treat deficiency
	Neuropathy	Vitamin B12 deficiency Pyridoxine deficiency Malnutrition Pressure neuropathy	Measure serum levels Nerve conduction study	Treat deficiency and malnutrition Cause is pressure neuropathy Consult neurologist
Muscle cramps	Latent tetany (Trousseau's sign, Chvostek's sign, lateral peroneal nerve tap sign)	Magnesium deficiency Calcium deficiency Alkalemia	Measure serum levels, may need to do magnesium load test	Treat deficiency
Numbness	Neuropathy	Malnutrition Deficiency of vitamin B12, pyridoxine Compression neuropathy	Physical examination Nerve conduction study	Treat specific cause
Causalgia (burning) pain	Neuropathy	Compression, alcohol, or diabetes	Physical examination Nerve conduction study	Pain can be treated with amitryptiline, dilantin, or carbamazepine

(cont.)

Table 5.3. (cont.)

Problem	Syndrome	Causes	Investigations	Treatment
Bone pains	Osteomalacia Osteoporosis Bone fracture	Causes of osteoporosis, osteomalacia is not caused by AN unless there is a concomitant cause of osteomalacia due to malnutrition; this is usually due to magnesium deficiency	Bone density For suspected stress fracture, the X-ray will likely be normal and a bone scan is then required to demonstrate the abnormality	Stress fractures should be treated with rest and investigation of osteoporosis or osteomalacia Refer to endocrinologist
	Extrapyramidal syndrome (EPS)	Major tranquilizers	Clinical examination	Stop or decrease dose For dystonia, intravenous or intramuscular antihistamine or benzatropine mesilate For other EPS, oral benzatropine mesilate
	Refeeding syndrome	Likely due to movement of potassium across cell membranes	Rule out other causes	Reassurance
	Serotonergic syndrome	Serotonin reuptake inhibitors	Physical examination Medication history	Stop serotonin reuptake inhibitors Have pharmacy check for drug interactions Symptomatic and supportive

Treatment

Treat the underlying cause.

Nursing implications

Ask questions to determine what the patient means by "aches and pains." If you suspect a drug side effect or interaction, then inform the physician or pharmacist as soon as possible.

5.3 Weakness

Case

A 30-year-old female who has had AN for 14 years complains of weakness. She has continued to have good exercise tolerance over the years despite continued low weight. Now she can no longer ride her bicycle or jog because of weakness. She thinks the weakness is caused by the disease, but she wonders whether there is anything she can do for it.

Comment

Weakness may be due to impaired muscle strength, early muscle fatigue, or limitation in exercise tolerance due to cardiac, respiratory, or deconditioning causes (Table 5.4). In AN, the most common causes of weakness are proximal myopathy due to potassium, magnesium, or phosphate deficiency, and decreased cardiovascular conditioning due to prolonged malnutrition. A history and physical examination should determine whether there is a specific muscle group that is weak (e.g. foot drop due to a compression neuropathy), proximal muscle weakness (potassium, magnesium, or phosphate deficiency), distal limb numbness (neuropathy), weakness brought on by repeated activity that recovers with rest (myasthenia gravis), increased jugular venous pressure (congestive heart failure), or shortness of breath and abnormal chest findings (aspiration pneumonia, lung abscess).

Nursing implications

- Prevent nerve compression of the lateral peroneal nerve where it crosses over the neck of the fibula, of the ulnar nerve where it crosses behind the elbow

Table 5.4. *Causes of weakness to consider in anorexia nervosa*

	Syndrome	Cause	Investigation	Comments
Muscle	Proximal myopathy	Deficiencies of potassium, magnesium, phosphorus, or selenium	Laboratory	Common
	Muscle fatigue with exercise	Myasthenia gravis	Edrophonium test (Tensilon)	Neurological consultation
Nerve	Distal symmetrical neuropathy	Deficiencies of vitamin B12 or pyridoxine, malnutrition	Nerve conduction study	Neurological consultation
	Single nerve affected	Usually compression but can be part of a mononeuritis multiplex (MNM) syndrome	Nerve conduction study to determine prognosis and time to recovery With MNM, investigation into the specific cause is necessary	Neurological consultation
	Non-specific pain over one or both upper outer thighs	Meralgia paresthetica due to compression of the lateral cutaneous nerve of the thigh	Clinical examination	Internal medicine or neurological consultation
Decreased cardio-respiratory fitness	Cardiomyopathy	Malnutrition Phosphate, selenium, thiamine, or vitamin B12 deficiency Valvular insufficiency	Echocardiogram Exercise stress test	Cardiology consultation
	Respiratory dysfunction	Respiratory muscle fatigue Pneumonia or lung abscess, empyema	Chest X-ray Pulmonary muscle function test	In AN, fever may not occur in infection Respiratory muscle function tests can be ordered as part of a pulmonary function test

(the funny bone), and of the radial nerve where it crosses behind the upper arm (Saturday night palsy) by providing soft mattresses and padding if the patient has a decreased level of consciousness. Remember that it may take six months or more to recover from a compression neuropathy.

- Report shortness of breath, paroxysmal nocturnal dyspnea, and orthopnea as soon as they occur. In AN, these can indicate acute life-threatening disease despite the patient being young.
- If the temperature is elevated above its previous level, even if it is less than 37 °C, this may represent a febrile response to infection. This may be the earliest indicator of pneumonia or other serious infection.

5.4 Confusion

Case

Two days after being hospitalized through the emergency department for an overdose, a 24-year-old female becomes agitated and confused. You are called by nursing staff because of her agitation.

Comment

A history and physical examination must be performed. Determine what medication(s) were taken in the overdose and what medications and intravenous fluids have been administered. Is there a history of alcoholism or illicit drug use? What observations has the nurse made?

The patient is probably suffering from an acute confusional state. The differential diagnosis includes an organic state due to focal or systemic cause and a functional state. The neurological examination will indicate whether there are focal neurological signs. If there are, then it must be presumed that there is a focal neurological cause. This would include central pontine myelolysis (decreasing level of consciousness), Wernicke's encephalopathy (nystagmus and ataxia), subdural causes (signs of head injury, the most common of which is simply a lump on the scalp), and focal seizure.

There are usually no focal signs.

An organic brain syndrome can occur with severe malnutrition in AN. It is often seen with very low total body fat or BMI of less than ten. The short-term memory impairment in the organic brain syndrome does not cause agitation or confusion. Therefore, there is something else happening in this case. The most important cause that must be ruled out immediately is hypoglycemia. Hypoglycemia occurs in AN because, with feeding, insulin is released to move glucose into the cells, but there is no liver glycogen to break down to prevent the glucose level from dropping afterwards. An immediate test of blood glucose must be performed: if the glucose is less than 2.5 mmol/l, administer 50 cm^3 of 50% dextrose in water intravenous push, followed by 100 mg of thiamine intravenously, 100 mg of thiamine intramuscularly, and an intravenous drip of 10% dextrose in water at 100 cm^3 per hour. The blood glucose must then be rechecked at that time and every hour until stable. Do not stop the intravenous glucose for a few days, and then only with blood glucose measurements four times a day.

Other causes of confusion include alcohol withdrawal, drug withdrawal, drug interactions or drug toxicity (e.g. malignant neuroleptic syndrome, serotonergic syndrome), hypomagnesemia, Wernicke's encephalopathy, infection, hyponatremia, and postictal state. Table 5.5 lists the common causes of confusion in eating disorders.

Nursing implications

- Report agitation and confusion as soon as they are noticed.
- Put on "close observation" protocol.
- Observe for any other physical signs.
- Ensure safety of the patient.

5.5 Loss of consciousness

Case

An 18-year-old female with a history of AN is brought to the emergency department having suffered a loss of consciousness. She is now awake. The casualty officer asks you to assess the patient.

Comment

First, clarify that the patient really did lose consciousness. If she did not, then the differential diagnosis is different and much broader. Episodes of loss of consciousness can be due to metabolic causes, seizures, decreased cerebral perfusion, and trauma.

Table 5.5. *Causes of confusion in eating disorder patients*

Focal neuro-logical signs	Cause	What to do	What to do next
Present	Postictal (focal seizure) Subdural Wernicke's encephalopathy Central pontine myelolysis	Full neurological examination as possible Feel cranium for lumps Avoid sedation or use of major tranquilizers	Neurological consultation for all patients with focal neurological findings
Absent	Alcohol withdrawal, drug withdrawal, drug interactions, drug toxicity (e.g. malignant neuroleptic syndrome, serotonin syndrome), hypomagnesemia, Wernicke's encephalopathy, infection, hyponatremia, postictal state	Observe level of consciousness Stop drugs that could be causative Administer thiamine 100 mg intramuscularly and intravenously Check blood sugar immediately and treat a blood sugar of less than 2.5 mm/l Do laboratory tests Remember normal temperature may be the only early indicator of infection	Observe carefully and treat the cause

Table 5.6. *Causes of loss of consciousness in eating disorder patients*

Type of cause	Cause	Investigations	Treatment
Metabolic	Hypoglycemia	Blood glucose	Thiamine, glucose
	Hyponatremia	Serum sodium	Slowly correct serum sodium and treat underlying cause
Cerebral hypoperfusion	Dysrhythmia	Cardiac monitor	Refer to cardiologist
Seizure	Medications, metabolic causes (hypoglycemia, hyponatremia, hypomagnesemia), decreased cerebral perfusion, focal or diffuse brain abnormalities	Laboratory Holter monitor Electroencephalogram Computerized tomography Medication record	Refer to neurologist
Head trauma	External trauma	Examine the head!	Refer to neurosurgeon

In AN, the most important causes to consider are hypoglycemia, seizures, and dysrhythmia. Hypoglycemia occurs because the liver has no glycogen left to form glucose when the blood glucose level drops. Seizures can occur due to medications or metabolic causes (hypoglycemia, hyponatremia, hypomagnesemia, decreased cerebral perfusion, alcohol or benzodiazepine withdrawal, or focal or diffuse brain abnormalities). However, an episode of loss of consciousness should be presumed to be due to dysrhythmia, and the patient should be monitored and risk factors should be sought. Trauma may be due to abuse or may be self-inflicted. Table 5.6 reviews the causes of loss of consciousness in eating disorders.

Nursing implications

- Measure blood sugar immediately on arrival.
- Treat according to the standard seizure protocol until the cause is clear.
- Attach a cardiac monitor and record any dysrhythmias.

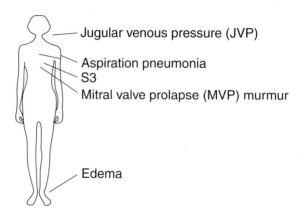

Figure 5.1. Causes of shortness of breath in anorexia nervosa.

5.6 Shortness of breath

Case

A 16-year-old female develops acute shortness of breath during an inpatient stay for the treatment of AN. A nurse telephones you to says the patient looks very ill.

Comment

It is likely that the patient has either aspirated her stomach contents or has gone into congestive heart failure due to hypophosphatemia (Figure 5.1). Both situations are potentially life-threatening.

As patients with AN become severely malnourished, their exercise tolerance will diminish gradually. However, if exercise tolerance worsens rapidly, or if this is associated with shortness of breath on exertion, then this indicates a significant abnormality usually associated with mineral deficiency and occasionally with decreased cardiac contractility. Under these circumstances, classical congestive heart failure may occur. The jugular venous pressure will be elevated; early on, however, there may be no crepitations but only some delayed expiration and wheeze (so called "cardiac asthma"). A chest X-ray will demonstrate pulmonary vascular redistribution but often little else. In the setting of AN, this is a life-threatening emergency and is almost always due to severe phosphate, potassium, or magnesium deficiency. In congestive heart failure, the shortness of breath will be made much worse by lying down or with any activity.

In aspiration pneumonia, the chest X-ray may be normal for up to 24 hours; the more severe the aspiration, the earlier changes will be apparent. If the patient has aspirated, then shortness of breath and often a dry cough will be evident. Localized dullness, crepitations, and rhonchi will be present early, before chest X-ray changes. Leukocytosis may take a day or two to develop, and there may be no fever. Table 5.7 lists the causes of shortness of breath in eating disorders.

Nursing implications

- Report the symptom, as it is potentially life-threatening
- Keep the patient on bedrest.
- Measure temperature, heart rate, and blood pressure, and auscultate the lungs and heart.

5.7 Chest pain

Case

A 30-year-old female with a 15-year history of AN complains of three months of chest pain that is increasing in frequency. She is worried that she is going to die of a heart attack. She asks your opinion.

Comment

AN is associated with an early onset of atherosclerosis. There have been several reported cases of patients dying from myocardial infarction. However, although up to 20% of patients with AN have typical or atypical angina, the prevalence of atherosclerosis is much lower. This could mean that the angina is due to coronary artery spasm, but this is not yet known.

First, take a history to determine whether the pain is anginal (a typical pain of heaviness felt usually in the mid chest, somewhere between the umbilicus and hard palate, precipitated by exercise or stress, and relieved by rest or nitrogly-cerine). Angina lasts at least one minute (usually at least five minutes) and never lasts more than 15–30 minutes (after which it would be a myocardial infarction). Usually, the pain suffered in AN is a chest-wall pain that is knife-like, lasts only a few seconds, and is worsened by touch. Other causes of chest pain are heartburn and esophageal spasm (this is just like angina but is not brought on or made worse by exercise and usually lasts many hours to a day). Finally, panic attacks may cause chest pain. See Table 5.8 for causes of chest pain in eating disorders.

Table 5.7. *Causes of shortness of breath in hospitalized patients with anorexia nervosa*

Problem	Syndrome	Cause	Investigation
Lung	Aspiration pneumonia	Aspiration of gastric contents	Clinical examination with a high index of suspicion; chest X-ray may be normal for first 24 hours
	Pneumonia, lung abscess, or empyema	Bacterial infection Poor response to bacterial infections in AN	Chest X-ray
Heart	Congestive heart failure	Hypophosphatemia	Chest X-ray
		Less likely low magnesium, low potassium, low thiamine, low selenium, protein-calorie malnutrition	Laboratory tests: phosphorus, magnesium, potassium, creatine phosphokinase
		Rarely, myocardial infarction will occur; this can occur by the age of 40 years in chronic AN	High index of suspicion for hypophosphatemia
	Dysrhythmia	Decreased perfusion and increased pulmonary pressure	Electrocardiogram

Table 5.8. *Causes of chest pain in eating disorder patients*

Organ	Syndrome	Cause	Investigation
Heart	Angina or atypical angina	Atherosclerosis or coronary artery spasm	Electrocardiogram during the pain Cardiological consultation
	Pericarditis	Inflammation of the pericardium	Electrocardiogram shows generalized ST segment elevation Echocardiogram shows increased fluid in the pericardium
Chest wall	Chest wall pain related to refeeding	Like the aches and pains of the refeeding syndrome	None
	Pathologic rib fracture (rib fracture that occurs from trauma that is normally insufficient to have caused it)	Osteomalacia Fractured ribs cause "pleuritic" chest pain, i.e. chest pain that is severe and knife-like and worsened by breathing	Rib fractures almost always occur due to osteomalacia Osteomalacia is not seen in AN unless there is a separate cause Refer to endocrinologist
Esophagus	Heartburn	Esophageal reflux Vomiting	History and trial of proton pump inhibitor, antacids, or prokinetic agent
	Esophagitis	Esophageal reflux Vomiting	History and trial of proton pump inhibitor, antacids, or prokinetic agent
	Esophageal spasm	Spasm of the esophageal muscle due to esophageal reflux	Pain like angina, but not precipitated or changed by exertion Relieved by nitroglycerine or calcium channel blockers

Nursing implications

- If the pain lasts for more than a minute, is felt deep in the chest, and is increased with activity, order an EKG and call the physician.
- If the patient's description of the pain sounds like heartburn, give 30 cm^3 of ward stock of antacid. If the pain is not relieved, call the physician.

5.8 Seizures

Case

The nurse finds an 18-year-old female with AN unconscious and with tonic–clonic movements. The movements have stopped, but the patient appears to be in a postictal state. You are called to see the patient.

Comment

Was it a seizure? There is always loss of consciousness with a generalized seizure. Therefore, if there was no loss of consciousness, it was not a seizure. It may have been a dystonic episode, carpopedal spasm, or decreased level of consciousness (same causes as for loss of consciousness).

If there was loss of consciousness with movement characteristic of a seizure, then the differential diagnosis would be seizure or pseudoseizure.

Pseudoseizures occur in patients who also have true seizures at least 30% of the time. Be careful not to conclude wrongly that a pseudoseizure is the cause of a clinical event in AN.

A pseudoseizure should be suspected if there is memory of the "seizure event" despite apparent unconsciousness during it, the events are atypical of seizures, typical post-seizure confusion and tiredness are absent, there is no change in the electroencephalogram (EEG) (30% of patients who have seizures have no seizure focus on the EEG, but there are non-specific changes that last for days after any generalized seizure), and there is absence of the normal marked postictal increase in prolactin. Table 5.9 lists the causes of seizures in eating disorder patients.

Nursing implications

- Check blood sugar.
- Record observations of seizure episode in detail.
- Routine seizure protocol.
- Check blood pressure and pulse rate and rhythm.
- Check for medication errors or medications taken by the patient themselves.

Table 5.9. *Causes of seizures in eating disorder patients*

Classification	Cause	Investigations	Special treatment
Metabolic	Hypoglycemia Alkalemia Hypomagnesesemia Hypocalcemia Hyponatremia	Blood glucose Screening bicarbonate Serum magnesium deficiency, calcium deficiency, sodium deficiency or rapid change in level	Correct abnormality Do not treat a single seizure with anti-seizure medications
Cerebral hypoperfusion	Dysrhythmia Vasovagal attack Postural hypotension	Postural blood pressure changes History of typical symptoms of vasovagal attack Holter monitor	Prevent cerebral hypoperfusion Cardiological consultation
Lowered seizure thresold	Medications (e.g. bupropion), medication withdrawal (e.g. benzodiazepines, barbiturates), alcohol withdrawal	Medication record	Benzodiazepines should be restarted and tapered at no more than 20% a day Alcohol withdrawal usually involves only one seizure so do not give anti-seizure medications

5.9 Palpitations

Case

A 17-year-old female AN admitted for feeding complains to you that she has noticed palpitations.

Comment

First, review the complaints to make sure that it is palpitations. Second, establish the clinical history of an episode:

- Was it of sudden or slow onset?
- Was it regular or irregular?
- How long did it last?
- Was it sudden or slow to go away?

Determine the pattern of the episodes:

- How many have there been?
- How often are they happening?
- Are they increasing in frequency?
- Do they seem to be brought on by stress, activity, purging, etc?
- Are there any other symptoms during the palpitations, such as chest pains or faintness?
- What do you do when they occur?

Palpitations are frequent in AN and most commonly occur after purging. The episodes are usually a few extra beats (may be from any cause), the sudden onset and offset of a rapid regular heart beat (usually paroxysmal atrial tachycardia), the slow onset of a rapid heart beat that goes away slowly (sinus tachycardia after stress, exercise, or purging), or at times the heart racing regularly and at times the heart going slowly (autonomic dysfunction). However, only the EKG recording can make the diagnosis of a dysrhythmia, so you must capture the palpitations, usually on a Holter monitor. If the palpitations are causing symptoms of faintness, loss of consciousness, chest pain, or seizure, then you must request an immediate cardiologist consultation because they may be caused by a life-threatening ventricular dysrhythmia (Table 5.10).

Nursing implications

- Monitor the patient carefully.
- Instruct the patient to lie in bed.
- Notify the physician.

Table 5.10. *Palpitations that need immediate cardiological consultation*

Symptoms of faintness, loss of consciousness, chest pain, or seizure with
  palpitation, anginal chest pains
Resting electrocardiogram shows runs of premature ventricular beats
  (PVB), more than five per minute PVB, PVB falls on down slope of T
  wave, abnormal site of pacemaker (not sinoatrial node), ST–T segments
  elevated more than 1 mm
Laboratory values: potassium less than 2.5 mmol/l, magnesium less than
  0.5 mmol/l

- Check apical heart rate, pulse rate, rhythm, and blood pressure.
- Take and record a history of the palpitations.

5.10 Bone fractures

Case

A 30-year-old female comes to clinic limping. She says she cannot walk on her
foot because it hurts. She wonders whether it is broken.

Comment

Progressive osteoporosis (decreased bone mass) occurs in AN. This predisposes, along with overexercise, to fractured bones. These usually cause stress
fractures of the feet, legs, or pelvis, compression fractures of the spine, causing
progressive and chronic pain, and fracture of the hip.

Osteomalacia (decreased bone mineral) can occur in AN, but it is not due
to protein-calorie malnutrition alone. There must be another cause, for which
an endocrine consultation will be required. Often, this relates to secondary
hypoparathyroidism due to chronic hypomagnesemia. Osteomalacia causes
other fractures, typically rib fractures, in AN.

Plan of action for the bones in anorexia nervosa

1. Prevention of osteoporosis:

   - nourish;
   - ensure adequate calcium intake (1500 mg a day in females);
   - ensure adequate vitamin D intake (400 IU a day);

- routine bone density scan in all patients with AN at onset of disease and at least every two years.

2. If bone density measurement shows osteoporosis range:

- same as for 1 above;
- measure body fat to assess nutritional status of body;
- if it is assumed that the patient is at a healthy weight range, but they are on the oral contraceptive pill or are not menstruating, then assess return of healthy weight (total body fat should be greater than 22%, or perform ultrasound of the ovaries to determine whether normal follicular development is occurring, which is evidence of normal endocrine status);
- order serum calcium, phosphorus, magnesium, and albumen;
- refer to osteoporosis clinic;
- consider use of biphosphonate.

3. If a bone pain has occurred that may be due to a fracture:

- obtain an X-ray;
- if the X-ray is negative, then there may be a stress fracture. Do a nuclear medicine bone scan (not density), which will demonstrate the stress fracture;
- consider orthopedic consultation;
- same as for 2 above.

Nursing implications

- Instruct the patient to rest the injured part.
- Reinforce the importance of taking vitamin D and calcium.
- Explain the bone density changes that occur in AN to the patient.

5.11 Rashes

Case

An emaciated 23-year-old patient presents with generalized itchiness of the skin, from which she has been unable to find relief. In your examination, you note enlargement of the gums, yellowing of the palms, downy hair growth on the back, and several oddly shaped scars on the forearms and thighs. What concerns would you have regarding this patient?

Comment

Skin signs (lanugo hair, hypercarotenemia) can help to make the diagnosis of AN and of associated behaviors such as purging (Russell's sign) or self-harm (slashing, burning, stabbing). Discussion of the skin findings in AN builds patient confidence in your expertise and helps to determine the risks of treatment (self-harm). It may also increase rapport, as the patient will usually accept treatment for physical complaints such as a rash.

Lanugo hair is diagnostic of AN. However, the reliability of the sign is not good, so it should simply be used as a reason for a high index of suspicion of AN. Hypercarotenemia is the yellowish skin color (without the occurrence of yellow eyes seen in jaundice) that occurs only in AN, hypothyroidism, and children who overeat carrots. Russell's sign is the scarring over the back of the hands that occurs if the hand is used forcefully and repeatedly in the mouth to induce vomiting. The dry and peeling skin over the palms and soles can be caused by zinc deficiency. If it is due to zinc deficiency, then it will normalize in about two weeks with zinc treatment (14–28 mg of elemental zinc or 100–200 mg of zinc gluconate a day for two months). Table 5.11 lists the rashes that are associated with eating disorders.

Nursing implications

- Inspect the skin for signs of self-harm and continue to search for and document any ongoing self-harm.
- Report any new rash to the physician.
- Use the treatment of any rash to build rapport. Patients are usually happy to receive advice and treatment of a rash.

5.12 Amenorrhea

Case

You see a 17-year-old female who is recovering from AN. She says that she is not menstruating and wonders when her menses will return.

Comment

Amenorrhea occurs at a body fat below 20% in most females who are not taking medications that induce menstruation (oral contraceptives). With weight regain, menstruation can return.

Important points

- Pregnancy can occur without menstrual periods (as long as ovulation is occurring).
- Females are usually not aware of whether they are ovulating.

Table 5.11. *Causes of rash in eating disorder patients*

Cause	Rash
Protein-calorie malnutrition	Lanugo hair Hypercarotenemia Edema (refeeding) Acrocyanosis Xerosis Pruritus
Nutritional deficiencies	Nail dystrophy Angular stomatitis Pellagra Acrodermatitis Scurvy Koilonychia
Behavioral	Dermatitis factitia Self-phlebotomy Self-harm
Case reports/rare associations	White dermographism Prurigo pigmentosa Pili torti Perniosis Neurofibromatosis
Purging behavior	Russell's sign Purpura Subconjunctival hemorrhage Edema Self-harm

- Menstruation may not start for up to 12 months after return of a healthy weight.
- Menstruation may not return at any time if severe stress or other factors that can cause amenorrhea occur.

Therefore, give your patients information about menstruation, ovulation, and the need for protection against pregnancy, even without menstruation, in AN.

Nursing implications

- Teach your patients.
- Ovulation, and pregnancy, can occur without menstruation.
- Females are usually not aware of whether they are ovulating.

- Menstruation may not start for up to 12 months after return of a healthy weight.
- Menstruation may not return at any time if severe stress or other factors that can cause amenorrhea are present.

5.13 Constipation

Case

Two weeks after being admitted for feeding, a 27-year-old female with AN says she has not had a bowel movement for the entire two weeks. She says you must do something now, because she is having severe intestinal cramps that increase each time she eats.

Comment

Common findings in AN include decreased food intake, decreased fluid intake, decreased fiber intake, history of laxative abuse, history of vomiting, weakness of the smooth muscle of the bowel, impaired peristalsis, decreased lower esophageal sphincter tone, impaired gastric emptying with associated early satiety, constipation, abdominal bloating, increased air swallowing, fecal impaction, and impaired recognition of the need to defecate.

- Assess and treat the reasons for constipation.
- Treat deficiencies of potassium and magnesium (they also cause the bowel to become weak).
- If there is paradoxical diarrhea (no stool, or pellet-like stools for several days, followed by watery diarrhea for a day or two, due to the non-absorbed fluid overflowing the blocking stool), give enemas to clear.
- Normalize the diet.
- Increase the fiber content (if you use too much fiber, the patient will have increased intestinal gas; if you use too little, it will not help).
- Make a plan with the patient to ingest at least 2 l of water (or other fluids acceptable to the dietician) a day.
- Use hydrophilic bulk-forming agents (see below).
- Use prokinetic agents (metoclopramide, domperidone).

If you doubt that there is still constipation, perform a plain X-ray of the bowel; some patients will continue to believe that they are constipated even when they are not.

Nursing implications

- Record time and observations of bowel movements.
- Ensure adequate fluid intake.
- Communicate with the pharmacist if a laxative withdrawal protocol has been ordered.

5.14 Abuse of laxatives, diuretics, diet pills, ipecac, and insulin

Patients with eating disorders (AN, BN) may misuse a variety of drugs in an attempt to promote weight loss by suppressing appetite, minimizing food absorption, eliminating fluid, or inducing vomiting. They may abuse laxatives, diuretics, diet pills, and/or ipecac. It has been estimated that nearly two-thirds of BN patients use laxatives and one-third use diuretics in an attempt to augment weight loss.

Laxatives

Some eating disorder patients ingest huge amounts of laxative drugs, many times in excess of the amount recommended by the manufacturer. Stimulant-type laxatives are used most frequently and are available in many over-the-counter preparations. Abuse of laxatives is not an effective method of weight loss, because the weight loss occurs predominantly due to transient loss of fluids or stool rather than prevention of calorie absorption. Furthermore, laxative use precipitates activation of the renin–angiotensin–aldosterone system and the secondary hyperaldosteronism subsequently promotes fluid retention. Chronic use of laxatives can result in serious sequelae, including loss of normal colonic peristalsis (laxative dependency) and cathartic colon (loss of normal colon function). This results in a potentially vicious cycle of further laxative abuse. Some patients also use enemas in an attempt to lose weight. Fleet enemas or tap-water enemas may be used as often as several times a week or even daily. See section 6.1 for a suggested laxative withdrawal protocol.

Diuretics

Diuretics are available in a wide variety of over-the-counter formulations for the treatment of premenstrual symptoms. They are used frequently in large quantities to promote weight loss. Diuretic use may begin as an attempt to control "edema," progressing to abuse with ingestion of diuretics in progressively larger quantities over time. As with laxative use, the initial diuretic use may promote secondary hyperaldosteronism and reflex fluid retention when diuretics are discontinued. Instead of allowing the system to readjust and fluid balance to be restored, the patient resumes diuretic use, believing that continued diuretic use is required to control the edema.

Patients may also abuse prescription diuretics. This is particularly common among health care workers who have access to such medications. Thiazide diuretics such as hydrocholorothiazine, loop diuretics such as furosemide, and potassium-sparing diuretics such as spironolactone and triameterene have all been described as drugs of abuse in eating disorder patients. Physicians should exercise caution in prescribing these medications for at-risk individuals, especially if the reason for the drug request is vague or poorly documented.

Ipecac

The relationship between ipecac and cardiomyopathy is less clear than thought previously. However, it is reasonable to instruct patients abusing ipecac that it has been reported to cause heart failure.

Ephedrine

Ephedrine is often used to cause weight loss. Sudden cessation of the drug, e.g. on hospitalization, can result in withdrawal symptoms. We recommend substituting dextroamphetamine for the ephedrine and tapering the dextroamphetamine.

Insulin

Diabetic patients may intentionally use too little insulin in an attempt to promote weight loss. This results in rapid progression of diabetic complications, including blindness and renal failure.

PART II

Treatment

Chapter 6
Principles of treatment

6.1 General principles of treatment

Eating disorders, like several other severe psychiatric illnesses, are seldom simply "cured." Relapses and a need for further treatment are common. Continued care and ongoing treatments that are lengthy and expensive are usually necessary for those with more chronic illness.

The eating disorder patient has the same right to treatment as patients with any other illness. They should not be denied this simply because their illness can be considered as "self-inflicted." Our society accepts that most illnesses are self-inflicted to some or other extent: malignant melanoma results from incautious exposure to the sun; cardiovascular disease is commonly associated with overindulgence in food; emphysema, lung cancer, and other neoplasias result from cigarette smoking; and HIV and AIDS are associated with unsafe sexual behavior and the use of contaminated needles. Where the eating disorder patient differs perhaps from the others is that the risk-taking behavior persists throughout the illness: if only the patient would change their behavior, then they would recover. However, it is not that simple. Once embarked on a course of illness, it is difficult to abandon it, particularly in the case of AN. There is something about the nature of being anorexic that is resistant to change. What makes anorexic behavior so persistent? That still needs explanation. Just as it was necessary to realize that nicotine is an extremely addictive drug before effective measures could be developed to help people give up cigarette smoking, so it will be necessary to understand what hold the eating disorder has on the patient before we can help them to recover from it.

The longer the patient has been caught up in the vicious cycle of their illness, the more difficult it is for them to renounce it. For that reason, early identification and intervention are important in order to prevent a spiral of ill health and unhealthy behaviors.

Because eating disorder sufferers have a right to treatment, they should receive the same sympathy and courtesy as other patients. A health professional has no more right to decline involvement with this illness than with any other. If the professional feels incompetent in treating eating disorder patients, then he or she should seek out ways to gain that competence. Medical educationalists need to teach students about eating disorders in the same way as they teach about other illnesses. The patient and their carers have a right to expect both sympathy and skill from their medical advisers and other health professionals in dealing with this illness.

It follows that issues of access are very important. At present, expertise (such as it is) is restricted largely to specialized centers. What is needed is a periphery of excellence, with ease of access to all who need it, and with the provision of information as to when medical help should be sought and where to go for it.

The severely ill patient is often patently irrational in their denial of illness, or at least their refusal of treatment. This occurs particularly in respect to serious AN. The question arises as to what extent the patient should be protected from themselves. As with other mental illnesses, there is a conflict between the preservation of the patient's human rights and the patient's right to receive the treatment that they need. The ways in which this conflict usually intrudes are as follows:

- The question of confidentiality. Patients in extreme physical danger because of their AN often refuse to grant health professionals permission to contact their relatives or friends. The health professional should use discretion in deciding whether to accept this limitation in just the same way as when judging what to do about suicidal intent.
- Involuntary treatment is sometimes necessary. As with all psychiatric illnesses, optimal practice is to use as little restriction or coercion as possible. However, the duty of care overrides this principle in times of extremity.
- Although coercion to accept measures to restore nutrition and to reverse medical complications is sometimes necessary and life-saving, it is not possible to coerce psychological changes. Hence, it is important that a therapeutic relationship remains intact.

Resources should be devoted to eating disorder treatment and research in direct proportion to its importance as a health problem. Unfortunately, this is not done, perhaps because it has not received strong advocacy from health professionals or in the community. The reasons for this, and ways to overcome the problem, need to be addressed.

6.2 Treatment of eating disorders not otherwise specified

Although patients with EDNOS are mentioned rarely in published reports about the treatment of eating disorders, the experience of specialist health professionals, general practitioners, and community support organizations is that these patients contribute a very large burden of psychopathology and considerable physical morbidity, particularly in the female population. Adolescent girls with weight problems leading to unhealthy eating behaviors, and those with low self-esteem and depressed mood, may go on to develop an eating disorder. Many may never fulfill the rather complex criteria for AN or BN but nevertheless have significant psychiatric and medical problems and fail to achieve their potential. Some women who have passed through a phase of AN in their youth may also have persistent problems. These may include overvalued ideas about weight and diet, erratic eating, self-esteem inappropriately dependent on their shape, depression, and physical problems resulting from their poor nutrition, such as osteoporosis and infertility.

6.3 Treatment of anorexia nervosa

The medical manifestations of AN that impair physical function and increase the likelihood of death must be treated, such as restoring normal electrolytes and treating severe anemia. Resistance to the treatment of medical complications is an indication for compulsory treatment. However, whether full nutritional restoration in hospital, psychotherapy, cognitive behavior therapy, or pharmacological intervention is actually beneficial for overall outcome remains unproven. Perhaps continued care, harm minimization, and prevention of complications while the disorder runs its course is the most important factor in management. Patients who stay in treatment and receive appropriate care tend to survive and eventually recover, at least partially, while those who fall out of treatment are at increased risk of mortality.

The medical manifestations need to be assessed and, where necessary, addressed. Abnormalities such as the down-regulation of thyroid hormone and the disturbed reproductive function are best considered as compensatory mechanisms to cope with the undernutrition, and their reversal is not indicated. However, other abnormalities, such as the disturbance of blood electrolytes, cardiac compromise, and hypothermia, require urgent correction.

The nutritional state needs to be restored, preferably by encouraging the patient to take a healthy normal diet with supplementation of some essential nutrients such as thiamine. If this cooperation cannot be achieved, then the use of special, energy-rich liquid diets or, if necessary, nasogastric feeding may be employed. Particular care needs to be taken during the early period of nutritional restoration because of the dangers of the refeeding syndrome. Electrolyte levels, particularly phosphates, must be monitored carefully and repeatedly.

Most clinicians incorporate some form of behavior therapy in feeding an emaciated patient. An operant conditioning behavioral program is recommended, but if used it should be of a lenient and flexible nature, with minimal restraint. It has been established that less restrictive behavioral approaches to the management of AN are more effective than those that are likely to be perceived by the patient as punitive and isolating. A more lenient approach is also likely to increase the effective participation by the patient in other aspects of treatment, such as psychotherapy.

Simultaneously, treatment of the psychiatric disorder is required. Various forms of psychotherapy are advised, particularly cognitive therapy, aimed at correcting faulty beliefs about food and weight and also at changing the characteristic ascetic, self-punitive, and self-denying value system from which the behaviors derive. Psychotropic medication is directed at the symptoms of depression and obsessionality, and may also be used to decrease the hyperactivity and restlessness that are often prominent.

Both physical and psychological treatments need to be administered in a setting in which the patient's behavior can be supervised. Firm boundaries need to be laid down; at the same time, reassurance, sympathy, and encouragement need to be given. Dedicated and skilled nursing staff and dietitians are invaluable in their day-to-day contact with patients. The treatment setting is often provided in a specialist inpatient ward, but the same effects can be achieved in a comprehensive and well-structured day program, or as an outpatient when there is a supportive home background and relatives or friends who are willing to work as cotherapists.

Different treatment modalities are recommended at different stages of illness and recovery. Specific treatments include nutritional rehabilitation, psychosocial interventions, and medications. However, no specific pharmacological or psychological interventions have proven to be effective. In some studies, particular modes of treatment in subgroups have been associated with better outcomes, e.g. family therapy in adolescents with AN. A recent trend is to orient therapy in accordance with the patient's motivation to change.

6.4 Treatment of the chronic patient: care versus cure

Much less attention has been given to the treatment of patients with chronic AN, which is widely misunderstood. It is important, as there are large numbers of chronic or partially recovered AN patients in the community. As in many illnesses, the rate of recovery is variable. The average patient with AN has evidence of the disorder for a few years, but many patients will continue to be anorexic for many years, some being anorexic for life. Health professionals may become confused when it appears that treatment does not work and may adopt a palliative care approach to the treatment of patients with "chronic" AN. This is tantamount to treating someone with asthma palliatively. A full understanding of this perspective results in the following conclusions in chronic AN:

- Treatment of intercurrent medical and psychiatric conditions is always indicated.
- The treatment of malnutrition continues, limited only by a continuing risk–benefit trade-off between the required nutritional goals and the patient's willingness to accept help.
- Focus on improved quality of life through rehabilitation.
- As in asthma, AN may remit at any time in its course.

All patients with AN can recover – and some recover decades into their illness. However, while the patient continues to suffer from chronic AN, the important mode of treatment is a rehabilitation model. Clinical remission in chronic AN sometimes occurs due to sociological change (e.g. divorce, death of a parent, decision to change careers) or because the patient simply becomes tired of being burdened with AN.

Patients with chronic AN have ongoing signs and symptoms of protein-calorie malnutrition. They will have thinning of their hair, dry and yellow skin, decreased ability to focus their eyes, shortness of breath on exertion, decreased exercise capacity, repeated dysrhythmias, dizziness on standing, weakness, tiredness, hypothermia, muscle cramps, and decreased memory and concentration. In addition, they will suffer from progressive osteopenia, leading eventually to osteoporosis, which will cause repeated fractures that start off as stress factors and later become symptomatic fractures of the spine and lower extremities. Controversy persists about the prevention of osteoporosis in this setting. The only measure known to be effective is full nutritional restoration. Supplementation of the diet with calcium or vitamin D should be used; bisphosphonates may be of benefit in patients in whom the advantages outweigh the risks. Hormone replacement therapy has been demonstrated to be ineffective.

Chronic AN is associated with social isolation, an inability to work and learn, and diminished functional activity, including with family and friends and at work. Depending on the level of debilitation of the patient, they may become reclusive, living in a small apartment and isolated from their family and friends. On the other hand, some chronic patients, although remaining thin and with significant weight and shape concerns, are integrated fully into their family, work, and society. Clearly, the goal of rehabilitation is to move a patient with AN from the former to the latter situation.

The overall goals in following a patient with anorexia are:

- To prevent death by monitoring depression, actively preventing suicide, building rapport, searching for psychological comorbidity that might prevent improvement or diminish quality of life, helping to set goals for rehabilitation, and continuing to celebrate life with the patient at every visit. This is the responsibility of all the health professionals involved in ongoing care.
- Medically, the frequency of follow-up varies, depending on the degree of illness, from every week to every three months. The weight, blood pressure, and heart rate should be taken. An inquiry regarding mood and plans should be taken, and goals should be established. If the patient is losing or gaining weight, then potassium, magnesium, and phosphate levels should be measured; if the weight is unchanged, this is not necessary. If there is significant deterioration in physical symptoms, then a systemic inquiry and physical examination with laboratory measures selected based on symptoms (often to include hemoglobin, electrolytes, creatinine, aspartate aminotransferase (AST), alkaline phosphatase, magnesium phosphate, vitamin B12, and ferretin) should be carried out.

The physician should concentrate first on physical complaints, since chronic anorexics find it much easier to talk about physical concerns. Treatment of physical problems is accepted easily and appreciated, and this increases rapport. Treatment of urinary incontinence (which commonly occurs in chronic AN), careful care of feet and toes, and prevention of osteopenia with calcium and vitamin D supplements should all be considered. Use of the oral contraceptive pill to continue menstruation and potentially to increase bone mass should be discussed. However, excessive attention to the medical treatment of osteopenia may be taken as a reason to focus less on renutrition, and hence may be counterproductive.

Psychologically, focus on rehabilitation and quality of life. Any comorbid condition such as a history of sexual abuse, substance abuse, or depression should be sought and may require long-term treatment before other psychological gains are possible. If motivational enhancement therapy is available, then patients should be encouraged to undertake it. A narrative approach is often used. This focuses on discussing the patient's life not according to their daily miseries but in the context of how someone would want to retell their story. The narrative approach should focus in particular on how their life could be improved to make the story more to the patient's liking. Often, it is useful to refocus the patient on their life by pretending it is a movie and changing the ending or episodes of the movie as they would if they were directing it.

One must be very careful regarding the involvement of the family in the treatment of chronic AN. There are often powerful feelings of guilt and anger that other family members hold towards the patient, and the patient may be ostracized from their family. Therefore, any discussions with family members are best done at the patient's request and with the patient present. Concrete issues should be given prominence. For example, the patient may wish to change their place of residence, apply for disability insurance, or discuss their place in the family. A health professional can act as a mediator for the patient and explain the patient's disease in the context of a process for which chronic rehabilitation is necessary.

It is of immense importance that the primary physicians respect the right of privacy of the patient. This is particularly difficult in the setting of a family physician who has treated the entire family for years. All patients who reach the age of majority should be treated as independent adults – regardless of their health or place of residence. All parties – the patient, their family, and other hospital staff – must be aware of this policy, otherwise patient confidentiality will likely be breached and the patient's trust lost forever. However, the responsibility of provision of care is always paramount, and if confidentiality must be broken to save life, then the issue must be dealt with openly and clearly.

6.5 Inpatient treatment

The primary goal of psychological treatment in inpatient management of AN is to assist in the process of weight gain and nutritional restoration. Behavioral approaches have been found to be the most appropriate psychological method for promoting weight gain on an inpatient unit. Bruch warned against the assumption that the restoration of weight gain in the short term was curative in AN. She suggested that behavioral programs had adverse effects in terms of the patient feeling out of control and would impair the patient's mood and self-esteem. Bruch highlighted that weight gain by behavioral principles is helpful only if it is part of an integrated inpatient treatment program that also focuses on other psychological issues. The clinician also needs to be aware of the potential iatrogenic dangers of refeeding using a behavioral program. There is absolutely no justification whatsoever for the implementation of harsh behavioral regimens to punish patients who are non-compliant with treatment.

Operant programs that are lenient have been found to be as effective as harsher programs in terms of weight gain and to be more effective in terms of compliance and acceptability to the patient. On one lenient program, patients had an initial week of bedrest and then were allowed free access around the unit and to visitors, contingent on gaining 1.5 kg in weight a week. If they did not gain this weight, they were placed on bedrest for a week or until the weight was gained. Investigating these types of programs, it was found that patients placed on bedrest programs found them necessary and helpful, with the worst implication of the programs being boredom. Evidence suggests that frequency of weighing of inpatients does not affect weight gain: patients being weighed three times a week gained as much weight as patients being weighed five times a week. As being weighed three times a week may act to reduce a patient's focus on weight, the authors recommended the lesser frequency of weighing.

If a more lenient program fails to promote weight gain, then it is suggested that brief reward programs be used. These programs are tailored more individually than the earliest operant programs. The goal is to gain 4–5 kg on the program, rather than the program being in operation for the entire admission. For a full description of brief reward programs, the reader is referred to the references list at the end of this book. However, the efficacy of these programs has not been evaluated.

6.6 Day-patient (partial hospitalization) treatment

Day-patient programs (also referred to as partial hospitalization programs) aim to contain the patient's eating disordered behavior and to facilitate weight gain on an intensive outpatient basis. Such programs attempt to balance intensive treatment of AN with maintaining the patient's connection with their psychosocial environment (family, friends, schoolwork). They also allow patients an opportunity to practice improved eating behaviors away from a hospital setting. An admission to a day program can be used following an inpatient admission (step down) or when progress in outpatient therapy is insufficient (step up).

Day programs have been reviewed in the international literature on eating disorders. The structure of day programs varies from institution to institution, but they typically run from three to seven days a week and follow cognitive-behavioral lines.

The term "day hospital" is generally defined as a facility that provides diagnostic and treatment services for patients who would otherwise receive traditional inpatient care. In addition to their use as an alternative to inpatient care, day hospitals also function as a transition from inpatient care to full-time life in the community and as an alternative to outpatient care.

Typically, inpatient and day-hospital programs have the same therapeutic goals and components. The primary difference between the two treatment approaches is that patients return to their homes at night and on weekends while attending a partial day-hospital program, rather than remaining at the hospital 24 hours per day. It should be noted that in partial day-hospital programs that provide treatment services on fewer than five days per week, patients are not provided structured treatment on the "off" days.

Despite the wide geographical differences, many commonalities exist among these programs. Specifically, similarities include the use of a multidisciplinary staff, reliance on group treatment as the primary means of therapy, inclusion of more advanced patients in the administration of treatment to newer patients, and the inclusion of the day program within a larger treatment model.

Day programs are seen as having a number of inherent advantages over the inpatient treatment of AN. First, day hospitalization allows the patient to maintain some social and vocational roles, thus encouraging more independence than inpatient treatment. Second, not removing patients from their natural environment is conducive to the generalization of therapeutic gains. Additionally, being at home for nights and weekends allows for greater family and peer contact and support. Intensive treatment in the community also allows exposure to the psychosocial situations that may have acted to play a role in maintaining the eating disordered behavior (family conflict, peer relations, eating at school, diet products being in the house, etc.). Repeated exposure to these situations allows the patient to develop alternative coping behaviors that can be developed and rehearsed within the group setting.

It is important to note several limitations: day programs provide less structure and greater patient freedom, and some patients may require a more structured inpatient environment. Due to the high level of commitment involved with day hospitalization, patients and their families have to be motivated and willing to devote the necessary time and effort. As a large portion of day treatment often occurs in a group setting, patients must demonstrate the ability to interact within a group. Serious medical complications, comorbid substance abuse, suicidal intent, or self-mutilation may warrant more intensive supervision or exclusion from day hospital treatment. The limited data on the outcome of patients treated in day programs indicate that programs with a significant cognitive-behavioral component have been reported to produce significant weight gain and improvement in both eating attitudes and psychosocial status. Cognitive-behavioral programs have been shown to be more effective than psychodynamically based programs.

Provision of day hospitalization for the treatment of eating disorders is an area that deserves more research. Specifically, more research is necessary regarding the clinical effectiveness and cost-effectiveness of these programs, especially over the long term. Although initial results appear encouraging, the ever-changing structure of the programs in addition to the mobility of patients within the different levels of care often complicate data collection. Future trends and program challenges appear to concentrate on trimming costs to maximize resources.

Summary

- Some patients with AN will benefit from an admission to a day program. Day programs are effective in achieving weight gain, modifying eating attitudes, and improving the psychosocial functioning of patients with AN.
- Day programs using cognitive-behavioral principles have been shown to be more effective than psychodynamically based programs – the least intrusive form of treatment that is clinically indicated should be used in the treatment of AN. As such, wherever possible, day programs should be used before an admission to an inpatient unit. Patients should be admitted to a day program following an inpatient admission to help the transition from hospital to home.
- The stage of AN needs to be kept in mind when making treatment decisions. The ability of a day program to treat patients at different stages of AN will depend on the intensity of treatment offered by a day program, e.g. it is recommended that a four-days-a-week program accept patients with a BMI above 16.

6.7 Indications for compulsory treatment

The following analogy may help to explain the need for compulsory treatment to an anorexic:

> If you knew a close friend was depressed – and if your friend asked you to let them commit suicide – would you? I think you would try to help them instead.

AN causes diminished decision-making ability. This being the case, physicians are absolutely obligated to protect patients with AN from harm, albeit frequently at odds with the delusional will of the patient. Around the world, countries recognize this fact and uphold the legal requirement for life-saving compulsory treatment in AN.

The regulations, laws, and methods of protection of patients with AN vary from country to country. The age of majority, the involvement of the family and the government, the role of social workers or other health care professionals, the need to report, the length of the committal, the rules regulating the review

Table 6.1. *Weighing the risks and benefits of treatment imposition*

Ideas in favor of imposed treatment	Ideas against imposed treatment
Patients' lives and health should be protected; death and suffering should be prevented	Patients are entitled to personal autonomy (freedom to choose their fate)
AN is a mental disorder that impairs judgment about treatment	AN is a sociopolitical phenomenon
Imposed treatment will bring about recovery or improvement	Imposed treatment will not lead to improvement and may cause harm

of committal, and even the rights and responsibilities of the treating physician vary between jurisdictions and must be clarified locally.

Resolving treatment refusal

- Seek to engage in a sincere and voluntary alliance.
- Identify the reasons for refusal.
- Provide careful explanations of treatment recommendations.
- Be prepared for negotiation.
- Promote autonomy.
- Weigh the risks versus the benefits of treatment imposition (Table 6.1).
- Avoid battles and scare tactics.
- Convey a balance of control versus non-control.
- Ensure that methods of treatment are not inherently punitive.
- Involve the family.
- Obtain ethical and legal clarification and support.
- Consider legal means of treatment imposition only when refusal is judged to constitute a serious risk.
- Consider a rehabilitation model of treatment in chronic AN.
- Conceptualize refusal/resistance as an evolutionary process.

Treatment refusal: factors to consider in decision-making

- Clinical decision analysis: estimate the risk of the alternative decisions.
- Beneficence: consider the benefits to the patient.
- Non-maleficence: avoid harm to the patient.
- Competence to consent to treatment: assess the patient's mental capacity for decision-making.

6.8 Common treatment problems

Problem 1: reaching agreement about admission to hospital

Case

A 21-year-old female with a five-year history of AN continued to express her motivation for recovery. However, all ten admissions over the past two years had ended with early discharge from hospital. Each time, discharge followed a disagreement (such as whether she would be allowed visitors and for how long, whether she would be able to eat food from the outside, how often she would be able to smoke cigarettes, the frequency of weighing, and the amount of sedation she could have). Subsequently, she was only admitted electively after a contract was formed and signed dealing with all of those issues that she agreed would be important to her.

Comment

Anorexic admissions are often highlighted in the memory of the staff by tremendous anxiety, splitting, and angry outbreaks, which reduce the likelihood of benefit. A contract, often reached only after weeks of negotiation, is the most effective method of reducing many of these difficulties. A copy of the contract should be retained by the patient, another by the team, and another put on the chart on admission.

Nursing implications

Review the contract to ensure that the treatment plan is consistent with it. If the patient requests something that is outlined in the contract, then refer to the contract and minimize other discussion around that topic.

Problem 2: exercise

Case

A 17-year-old female anorexic has a history of extreme exercise for many hours a day. She says she does not think she can stop exercising in hospital. Before hospitalization, guidelines are given, including no passes for one week, or longer if adequate weight gain is not achieved, standard ward yoga once a week, sedation, and anxiety-reduction techniques. After admission, the patient does not gain weight. She is suspected of exercising in the shower seven times a day and running on the spot in her room; she is always moving about on the ward and never sits still. As a result, her showers are reduced to four times a day, her door must be left open unless approved temporarily by her nurse, and she is told her sedation will continue to be increased until she can rest on her bed.

Comment

The patient must be supported in finding methods of normalizing exercise. However, it is better to base the plan on successful weight gain rather than reduced exercise. Explain to the patient that exercise is a good thing – but just like anything in life, too much is not good. Explain osteoporosis, muscle wasting, and the horrid outcome of anorexia after 20–30 years. The authors employ an exercise manual that their occupational therapist uses to gradually increase exercise. They have demonstrated that this increases satisfaction about exercise and does not decrease the rate of weight gain.

Nursing implications

Review the plan regarding exercise. If the patient is exercising outside the guidelines, they should be reminded and stopped. If they are exercising within the guidelines but excessively, then the guidelines will have to be revised. Use techniques to reduce anxiety in order to help the patient cope with not exercising.

Problem 3: using a Ulysses agreement

Case

A 23-year-old anorexic has been certified three times over the past year for extreme weight loss that resulted in an organic brain syndrome and hypoglycemia. Each time, as her weight drops, her insight has diminished. After the next admission, with the patient recovered enough to have improved cognition, a contract is signed that sets out the circumstances under which she should be readmitted to hospital to avoid certification. Using the contract, she receives refeeding early and requires only a brief admission.

Comment

The Ulysses agreement permits planning and consensus and often improves understanding. While developing the agreement, the patient often shares and explains their fears.

Nursing implications

The Ulysses agreement is a contract specifying the conditions under which the patient agrees that they will need further treatment. It often takes a number of sessions to achieve, and is best reached by an interested social worker.

Chapter 7
Medical and nutritional therapy

7.1 Medical treatment

The physical manifestations of eating disorders result from malnutrition, the pathophysiologic consequences of malnutrition, behaviors used to cause weight loss, self-injurious behaviors, and iatrogenic causes. Table 7.1 lists some of the physical complications of eating disorders that require specific treatment, while Table 7.2 lists those for which no specific treatment exists. Algorithms for the management of patients with AN and BN by a primary physician are shown in Figures 7.1 and 7.2, respectively.

Medical goals of therapy

- To assess and treat coexistent nutritional deficiencies.
- To uncover comorbid physical conditions (e.g. hyperthyroidism).
- To assess and treat the effects of malnutrition (e.g. osteoporosis).
- To develop healthy eating habits.
- To treat binge and purge behavior.
- To achieve a healthy weight (total body fat).
- To uncover and treat complications (e.g. erosion of teeth) of behaviors being used to cause weight loss.
- To recognize and seek treatment for self-injury (e.g. bruising, self-phlebotomy).
- To prevent, diagnose, and treat complications of treatment (e.g. habituation to anxiolytics).

Beginning treatment

- Build rapport and develop a therapeutic alliance.
- Family involvement and treatment should be started.

128

Table 7.1. *Physical complications of eating disorders for which there are specific treatments*

Physical complication	Cause
Sores at sides of mouth	Riboflavin deficiency
Bleeding, friable gums	Scurvy
Dry skin, especially on palms of hands and soles of feet	Zinc deficiency
Nystagmus or ophthalmoplegia	Wernicke's encephalopathy
Confusion or forgetfulness	Drug toxicity; low serum sodium, magnesium, phosphate, vitamin B12, glucose, or thiamine deficiency
Symmetrical proximal weakness	Magnesium, potassium, phosphate, or calcium deficiency
Seizures	Hypoglycemia, drug withdrawal, drug toxicity, hypomagnesemia, dysrhythmia
Loss of consciousness or coma	Hypoglycemia, overdose, Wernicke's encephalopathy, severe hyponatremia, central pontine myelolysis
Latent tetany with a Chvostek's, Trousseau's, or lateral peroneal nerve tap sign	Magnesium deficiency, less likely potassium deficiency, alkalemia
Causalgia (intense burning feeling)	Peripheral neuropathy (alcohol, diabetes mellitus, recovering compression neuropathy are the most common causes)
Decreased sensation, peripheral neuropathy	Vitamin B12 deficiency, thiamine deficiency, malnutrition, pressure neuropathy
Foot drop	Nerve compression of lateral peroneal nerve
Mitral valve prolapse murmur	Normally present in 17% of healthy young females; worsens with weight loss improves with weight gain. If associated with the murmur of mitral regurgitation, can predispose to dysrhythmia and bacterial endocarditis
Dysrhythmias	Low potassium, magnesium, or calcium, autonomic dysfunction, QT prolongation, volume depletion, coexistent hyperthyroidism

(cont.)

Table 7.1. (cont.)

Physical complication	Cause
Postural hypotension	Volume depletion
Pitting edema	Refeeding syndrome, hypoalbuminemia
Abdominal tenderness	Obstipation, superior mesenteric artery syndrome, pancreatitis
Bone pain	Fracture, stress fracture, osteomalacia

Table 7.2. *Physical complications of eating disorders for which there are no specific treatments – only feeding*

Physical complication	Cause
Generalized alopecia	Severe malnutrition; will reverse with recovery
Aphthous ulcers	Usually no specific cause
Erosion of teeth, gingivitis	Purging
Swelling of sides of face	Can be due to purging and malnutrition independent of purging
	Stop purging, hydrate, use the sucking of lemons and warming (increases parasympathetic tone)
Lanugo hair	Reverses with weight restoration
Hypercarotenemia	Due to slow metabolism of carotene
	Of no pathological consequence
	Reverses with recovery
Russell's sign	Scarring over the back of the hand due to habitual pressure on the teeth while purging
	No treatment
Acrocyanosis	Warm and volume replete

- Set progressive nutritional goals.
- Exercise should be limited.
- Binge and purge behavior should be monitored and goals for normalization set.
- Tapering of laxative abuse should be encouraged and managed with a suggested protocol (Table 7.3).

Weight loss and malnutrition should be prevented by early diagnosis and treatment. When rapid weight loss has occurred or when body weight is extremely low, medical instability and death can result. Recurrent vomiting,

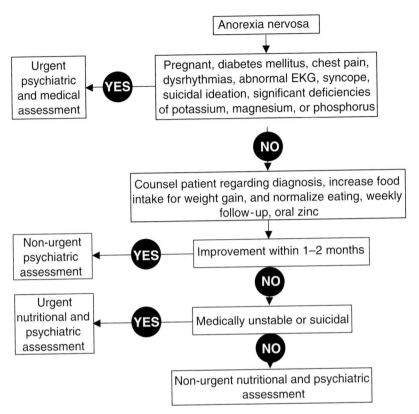

Figure 7.1. Management of anorexia nervosa.
Reprinted with permission from Birmingham, C. and Goldner, E. Eating disorders. In: Canadian Pharmaceutical Association (ed.) *Therapeutic Choices*, 3rd ed. Ottawa: Canadian Pharmaceutical Association, 2000, pp. 836–42.

misuse of laxatives, enemas, suppositories, diuretics, ipecac, self-phlebotomy, or gavage, overexercise, and underuse of insulin in insulin-dependent diabetics can lead to volume depletion, electrolyte abnormalities, vitamin and mineral deficiencies, and organ dysfunction. Signs and symptoms that indicate medical instability and should prompt full medical assessment are shown in Table 7.4.

If medical instability is present, then stabilization is begun through bedrest, intravenous fluid, and correction of any deficiencies. Routine administration of multivitamins, thiamine, phosphorus, and potassium is mandatory. Feeding may exacerbate deficiencies as a result of the movement of electrolytes, vitamins, and minerals into cells and between fluid compartments. Thus, volume, electrolytes, and minerals repletion must precede refeeding (see Section 7.3). Reassessment of potassium, magnesium, and phosphorus should be made

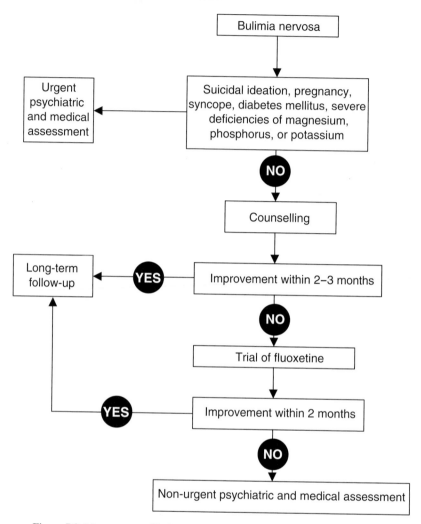

Figure 7.2. Management of bulimia nervosa.
Reprinted with permission from Birmingham, C. and Goldner, E. Eating disorders. In: Canadian Pharmaceutical Association (ed.). *Therapeutic Choices*, 3rd ed. Ottawa: Canadian Pharmaceutical Association, 2000, pp. 836–42.

routinely, daily for the first week and then three times a week. When required, the type of intravenous fluids given should be assessed individually, but commonly 0.9% normal saline is given for fluid repletion. Dextrose should not be given as it can precipitate an acute thiamine deficiency, resulting in Wernicke's encephalopathy. Once thiamine has been administered, 5% dextrose in 0.9% saline, or 3.3% dextrose in 0.3% saline, can be administered, if required. The

Table 7.3. *Laxative withdrawal protocol*

Step I

1. Discontinue all stimulant laxatives.
2. Initiate docusate 200 mg orally three times daily (increase to 200 mg orally four times daily as tolerated).
3. Initiate psyllium hydrophilic muciloid 5 g orally daily to three times daily (as tolerated).
4. Initiate fruit-based laxative 30 cm^3 orally daily to three times daily (as tolerated).
5. Initiate magnesium hydroxide/cascara combination orally daily as follows:

   - Magnesium hydroxide 30 ml/cascara 30 ml for previous laxative use of less than 20 bisacodyl 5-mg tablets or equivalent per day.
   - Magnesium hydroxide 45 ml/cascara 45 ml for previous laxative use of 20–40 bisacodyl 5-mg tablets or equivalent per day.
   - Magnesium hydroxide 60 ml/cascara 60 ml for previous laxative use of 40–60 bisacodyl 5-mg tablets or equivalent per day.
   - Magnesium hydroxide 90 ml/cascara 90 ml for previous laxative use of more than 60 bisacodyl 5-mg tablets or equivalent per day.

   These are recommended guidelines only. Because of variation in individual response, increase the magnesium hydroxide/cascara dose by 10 ml (i.e. 5 ml each) every two days until bowel movement occurs.
6. Ensure adequate water intake.

Step II

1. Taper magnesium hydroxide/cascara dose (based on response/symptoms*) by 5 ml orally every three to seven days until no longer needed.
2. If no bowel movement for more than 5 days, increase magnesium hydroxide/cascara dose back to the previous level where bowel movement was adequate.
3. If no bowel movement for more than 7 days, continue with current magnesium hydroxide/cascara dose and add bisacodyl 15 mg orally as per bowel retraining protocol. Follow protocol until bowel movement.

General guidelines

1. Before implementing each step, monitor for bowel movements, bowel sounds, and/or flatulence. If patient does not have a bowel movement for five to seven days, palpate all four quadrants to ensure no obstruction.
2. Encourage patient to:

   - increase fiber and water intake;
   - resist the temptation to take other laxatives without consulting staff.

(cont.)

Table 7.3. (cont.)

3. Advise the patient that during the early stage of treatment:

- the feelings of bloating, fullness, and constipation are common until normal peristalsis and bowel habit return;
- edema is common and is related to the degree of dehydration before treatment. It will resolve after 5–14 days. Ask the patient to elevate their limbs and decrease salt intake if edema is bothersome.

4. Reiterate the danger of laxative abuse:

- electrolyte disturbances may lead to muscle weakness, renal impairment, and, most importantly, life-threatening arrhythmia or sudden death;
- cathartic colon (bowel will not work on its own);
- reflex constipation (will need to consume more and more laxatives due to increasing tolerance).

*Recommended rate of tapering only. Hold dose if patient has diarrhea. Slow down tapering if patient is complaining of constipation.

administration of glucose is necessary if hypoglycemia occurs during feeding; this may happen because the pancreas begins to release more insulin in response to feeding, but when the blood glucose falls there is insufficient carbohydrate stored in the liver to maintain a safe blood glucose level (greater than 2.5 mmol/l). If renal function is impaired or if the patient has not passed urine, then potassium should not be administered in order to prevent hyperkalemia. Potassium can be started once the patient begins urinating.

Cardiac chest pain (see Section 4.5) or dysrhythmia should prompt immediate investigation. If there are frequent ventricular premature beats, a prolonged QT interval (greater than 450 ms or an increase of 60 ms beyond baseline EKG) occurs with severe hypokalemia, hypomagnesemia, or hypophosphatemia, then cardiac monitoring should be considered. Depending on the expertise of the general practitioner, patients who have dysrhythmias associated with symptoms including syncope, collapse, and typical or atypical angina should be referred to a specialist.

The nutritional repletion that follows initial stabilization should begin slowly and should be monitored carefully.

Hospital treatment for the medically unstable patient

- Bedrest.
- Intravenous fluids and minerals as necessary.

Table 7.4. *Indicators for admission to hospital*

Concern	Criteria for admission
Weight loss	Rapid (more than 4 kg over one month)
	Inability to eat or keep anything down
Neurologic	Confusion, syncope, decreased level of consciousness, loss of consciousness
	Confusion, organic brain syndrome
	Ophthalmoplegia, seizure, tetany, ataxia
Cardiac	Dysrhythmia that causes symptoms more than palpitations, or any dysrhythmia of ventricular origin
	Abnormal pacemaker
	QTc greater than 450 ms
	Signs of severe autonomic dysfunction (as read by cardiologist on Holter monitor)
Metabolic	Renal failure with increasing creatinine or urine output less than 400 cm^3/day (oliguria), serum sodium less than 125 mmol/l, potassium less than 2.5 mmol/l, hypoglycemia (blood glucose less than 2.5 mmol/l), hypophosphatemia (phosphorus below normal on fasting sample), magnesium less than 0.55 mmol/l (normal above 0.7 mmol/l)
Muscular	Rapidly diminishing exercise tolerance (due to muscular weakness not accounted for by a metabolic abnormality or diaphragmatic wasting)
Pregnancy	Fetus is at risk
Diabetes	Blood glucose control almost always requires inpatient admission to control eating behavior, activity, and insulin without putting the patient at risk

- Correction of deficiencies.
- Only after deficiencies are corrected and volume restored should refeeding begin.
- Begin refeeding slowly to avoid the refeeding syndrome (unmasking latent deficiencies with a load of macronutrients (carbohydrates, fats, proteins)).
- The preferred feeding method is meal support with meals designed by a dietitian in conjunction with the patient. Meals are usually begun at about 1200 calories a day. If the patient is unable to eat, then use supplements, behavioral strategies, or nasogastric feeding.
- During refeeding, supplements of thiamine 100 mg for five days, multi-vitamins daily, potassium chloride 20 mEq twice a day, phosphorus 500 mg twice a day, and zinc gluconate or sulphate, with 14–28 mg of elemental zinc daily (100–200 mg of zinc gluconate), should be given. Monitor potassium,

phosphorus, and magnesium daily for five to seven days, and then three times a week.
- Table 7.5 presents a schema for admitting a physically ill eating disorder patient to hospital.

Caution

- Hypoglycemia can occur during refeeding when insulin has been stimulated by food intake but there is a lack of liver glycogen to respond to a drop in blood sugar.
- Hypophosphatemia can occur rapidly. If the phosphate level drops, then the amount of oral supplementation should be increased and the level measured at least once daily. If the level continues to drop, then discontinue all feeding and give oral and intravenous phosphate.
- Hyponatremia (serum sodium lower than 125 mmol/l) must be corrected slowly, otherwise cerebral edema can occur, with decreased level of consciousness and even central pontine myelolysis.

Medications

Prokinetic medications

Domperidone or metoclopramide are useful in treating early satiety, abdominal discomfort, and esophageal reflux. The dose may be varied from 5 to 20 mg as required. The medication should be given half an hour before meals. Both drugs have the potential for the extrapyramidal side effects of the major tranquilizers. However, only a small amount of domperidone crosses the blood–brain barrier, so it is much less likely to cause central side effects.

Bulk-forming agents

Bulk-forming agents for the bowel, which bind water to help normalize bowel function, should be used routinely. Docusate sodium, psyllium (hydrophilic mucilloid), or similar agents should be prescribed daily with adequate fluid intake (at least 2 l a day).

Anxiolytics

Anxiolytics such as clonazepam, diazepam, and lorazepam may be used, but they can cause amnesia, reduced emotional control, and habituation. Clonazepam can be started at 0.5 mg twice a day. Titrate upwards every two or three days to the required effect. The maximum dose of clonazepam is 20 mg a day.

Table 7.5. *Suggested schema for inpatient orders*

Encourage rest. Specify limitations to activity, e.g. wheelchair only, no physical activity, no passes off the ward.

Dietician to order diet.

Admission laboratory work:

- hemoglobin, white blood cell count, platelets, serum sodium, potassium, chloride, bicarbonate, blood urea nitrogen, creatinine, aspartate transaminase, alkaline phosphatase, magnesium, calcium, phosphorus, ferritin, vitamin B12, red blood cell folate, zinc, international normalized ratio (INR)
- electrocardiogram
- urinalysis (midstream urine).

Hypnotic as required: zoplicone 7.5–15 mg at bedtime, or chloral hydrate 500–1000 mg at bedtime, or trazodone 25–50 mg at bedtime, or clonazepam 0.5–2.0 mg at bedtime.

Anxiolytic (beware the amnestic and disinhibiting effects of benzodiazepines):

- lorazepam 0.5–2.0 mg sublingually up to every hour as required
- clonazepam 0.5–2.0 mg orally twice a day.
- Routine blood work: potassium, phosphorus, and magnesium daily for seven days and then every Monday, Wednesday, and Friday. Daily bloodwork should be continued or restarted if there is a deficiency of any of these three minerals.

Standard supplements:

- potassium chloride (pills, effervescent, or liquid) 24 mEq three times a day for 21 days
- sodium phosphate solution 5 ml (550 mg of phosphorus) three times a day for 21 days. Continue once a day if weight gain continues at a rate greater than 0.5 kg a week
- multivitamins two tablets a day for two months and then one tablet a day
- thiamine 100 mg a day for five days
- zinc gluconate 100 mg daily for two months.

Intravenous rehydration if required: give normal saline (0.9% NaCl solution) at 100–150 cm^3 per hour until intravascular volume is normalized based on jugular venous pressure and postural blood pressure.

Bowel routine:

- sodium dioctylsulfasuccinate 200 mg twice a day for two months or longer
- give 15–30 cm^3 of magnesium sulfate and 15–30 cm^3 of cascara every seven days if required for severe constipation. If this is required or there is a history of bowel complaints, consult pharmacist to order the bowel retraining protocol (see Section 4.6)
- domperidone or metoclopramide 5–20 mg half an hour before meals (three times a day) and at bedtime. Titrate dose upward in 5 mg increments. Use domperidone in preference to metoclopramide, which is more likely to cause extrapyramidal side effects.

Antidepressants

The major indication for antidepressants is in the treatment of coexistent major depression. A minor indication is the treatment of bingeing and purging behavior. Serotonin reuptake inhibitors are the preferred antidepressants in eating disorders, because of their efficacy and reduced cardio- and neurotoxicity. They can be used to treat major depression, binge–purge behavior, and coexistent obsessive-compulsive disorder. Do not use tricyclic antidepressants or monoaminoxidase inhibitors because of their potential toxicity. Do not use bupropion because of the risk of seizures.

Cyproheptadine

This can be used to facilitate weight gain. The only patients who are willing to take it are chronic AN who desire the increased quality of life associated with modest weight gain. It should be started at bedtime, as it is sedating, beginning with a dose of 4 mg and increasing as required and if tolerated to 16 mg.

Major tranquilizers

The major tranquilizers olanzapine, chlorpromazine, and loxapine can be used to treat AN patients whose disorder is severe and entrenched or in whom the degree of obsessionality is nearly psychotic in degree. Monitor for extrapyramidal side effects, and either adjust the dose downward or discontinue drug if they occur. Only olanzapine appears to reduce anorexic ruminative thinking.

Zinc

Zinc supplementation increases the rate of weight gain irrespective of serum zinc level. Oral zinc should be given in a dose of 14–28 mg of elemental zinc (100–200 mg of zinc gluconate) a day. Zinc causes gastric upset in about 2% of patients; this is reduced by taking it with meals.

Ondansetron

Ondansetron has not been shown to be useful in preventing purging.

Notes

- Normalization of body fat is necessary for psychological or medication therapy to be optimally effective.
- The response of individual patients to an antidepressant is variable. Lack of success or side effects with one antidepressant should be followed by sequential trials of other antidepressants.

Table 7.6. *Pharmacological risks*

Drug	Risks
Cisapride	Can lead to prolongation of the QT interval and sudden death
	Has been removed from the market in most countries and should not be used
Bupropion	Can cause seizures in eating disorders
Serotonin reuptake inhibitors	Can lead to serotoninergic syndrome if given in excessive doses, or combined, or if metabolism is reduced due to drug interactions
Major tranquilizers and addition of medications with the properties of major tranquilizers, including prokinetic agents (domperidone, metoclo-pramide, trilafon)	Extrapyramidal side effects: acute dystonia, tardive dyskinesia, akathesia, parkinsonism, malignant neuroleptic syndrome
Herbal remedies	May have the properties of laxatives, diuretics, steroids, and other active agents
Stimulants (e.g. ephedrine) (may be used covertly to promote weight loss)	Can lower the thresold to seizures and dysrhythmia and can result in withdrawal symptoms if stopped suddenly
Benzodiazepines	To avoid symptoms of withdrawal, including seizures, taper no faster than 20% a day
Alcohol	Beware of alcohol withdrawal
Habituation	Beware of addiction in patients with history of addictive behavior
Overdose	Many patients with AN will stockpile drugs
	Monitor medication use, multi-doctoring, and drug hoarding

- In AN, the total body fat mass is low, the lean body mass is more nearly normal, the renal and liver function are usually normal, and the metabolic rate is often high. The volume of distribution of drugs and the dose of drugs required are often as high as, or higher than, those in normal-weight patients.
- Consideration should be given to the effect of any medication on cardiac function. Any agents that prolong the QT interval should be avoided, or the EKG should be reassessed during their use.
- Risks associated with medications used in eating disorders are listed in Table 7.6.

7.2 Nutrition: an overview

Serum levels of nutrients are a poor measure of their stores in the body. The body adapts to a reduced caloric intake by lowering the metabolic rate, reducing the use of nutrients, and forming a new equilibrium between serum levels and stores. Feeding rapidly increases the metabolic rate and the rate of use of nutrients, uncovering deficiencies and leading to morbidity and sometimes death.

Nutrition is the state of the nutrients of the body. It includes the seeking, intake, digestion, absorption, transport, storage, and use of nutrients. Nutrients are categorized as macronutrients and micronutrients. Macronutrients are the carbohydrates, fats, and proteins. Micronutrients are the vitamins and minerals. Vitamins and minerals are found in the body in small amounts. They are transported (often bound to proteins for transport purposes) to the organs and cells that they help to function; sometimes, there is a storage depot (e.g. vitamin B12 usually has a three- to five-year store in the liver). The different nutrients have differences in food source, quantity in the diet, digestibility by the body, absorption, method of transport, amount that is stored, other nutrients or factors that are required to function properly, and daily requirements in health and disease.

Energy

The energy needed for the body to function is provided by nutrition. More than 90% of the available energy is stored in adipose tissue. The rest is in a small amount of carbohydrate (glycogen) in the liver and muscle (Figure 7.3).

Protein-energy malnutrition

When the body takes in less energy than it needs, stored energy is used. All tissues of the body need glucose for energy. Only the brain after a day or so of starvation can then use ketone bodies for energy. As the blood glucose falls, so insulin falls, glucagon rises, and later cortisol and catecholamines rise. This results in the breakdown of liver glycogen, a store of carbohydrate, with the subsequent release of glucose into the blood. Liver glycogen normally lasts for a day. In the presence of underlying starvation or liver dysfunction, and in children, the carbohydrate will run out sooner. Next, the body uses the glucose produced from fat. Adipose tissue stores of fat break down, releasing free fatty acids into the blood. These are converted to glucose and ketone bodies by the liver. Stores of fat can last from days to weeks. Next, protein, particularly from muscle, breaks down, releasing amino acids into the blood, which are converted to glucose by the liver.

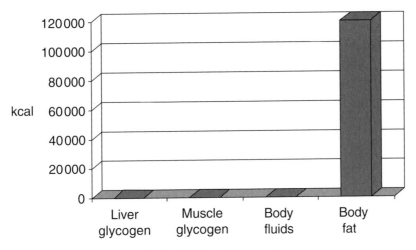

Figure 7.3. The body's usable stores of energy.

With starvation, carbohydrate (glycogen) stores are used first, followed by adipose tissue (fat), and then protein (amino acids). Once fat is broken down, ketone bodies rise in the blood, causing mild acidemia. In about 2% of patients, starvation ketosis results in a severe progressive acidemia; in other patients, the acidemia is mild and accompanied by a drop in bicarbonate of just a few millimoles. Ketone bodies are osmotically active and carry water from the body through the kidney, along with minerals. Protein loss causes wasting of the muscles of the body, including the respiratory muscles.

Most patients with AN, irrespective of their severe malnutrition (marasmus), have normal serum albumen. Some patients, however, develop low albumen, a fatty liver, and the edematous bloated picture that one recognizes from the pictures of Africa's starving children. Even a minimal intake of energy and protein in the diet is enough to prevent hypoalbuminemia and low protein malnutrition (kwashiorkor). Thus, low albumen indicates more severe malnutrition and should be treated with a high-protein diet. A high-protein diet should contain 1.5 rather than 0.7–1.0 g of protein per kilogram of body weight per day.

Understanding nutritional deficiencies

It is perhaps easiest to understand nutritional deficiencies by the analogy of a university student's struggle with money. Think of a nutrient in the body as money, the money in the bank as the nutrient stored, the pocket money as the serum level, and daily spending as the physiological function of the nutrient. At the beginning of their studies, a student has money in the bank, money in their pocket, a car, an apartment, and money for fun. As time goes by, the money in the bank goes first. They still have money in their pocket, although perhaps their activities are limited. Next, they may have to sell the car. Gradually, their possessions diminish, until finally they are left with a little money in their pocket, a little in the bank, no car, no outings, and a shared room at the dorm. Notice that the tissue levels (the bank) fell during the whole process, the serum levels (the pocket change) reflected poorly the wealth of the student, and the loss of possessions happened suddenly at points along the way.

It is the same with nutrients. Serum levels often fall very late in the course of a deficiency. Measures of total body nutrients, if available, are better indicators of nutritional status. Organ damage can occur suddenly and without warning symptoms. Details of important deficiency states are listed in Table 7.7.

Electrolyte disturbance typically takes the form of a hypokalemic, hypochloremic metabolic alkalosis. Severe potassium depletion is associated with muscular weakness and cardiac arrhythmias, but potassium should be given carefully because it may rise too rapidly if there is coexistent dehydration. Importantly, the serum creatinine may be normal in the face of renal failure. This is because the serum creatinine is proportional to body muscle – which is low. Thus, the serum creatinine should be below normal; if normal, it would indicate significant renal dysfunction.

Once an electrolyte abnormality is found, others are likely to emerge. However, because of the very unusual premorbid diets of patients, unusual deficiencies, such as copper deficiency, occur. Hypomagnesemia is common. The complaints of muscle weakness, cramping of the leg muscles at night, difficulty in maintaining visual focus for more than 30 minutes, and impaired short-term memory are typical of total body magnesium deficiency. Magnesium deficiency impairs kidney retention of potassium. This should be suspected if low potassium does not correct with supplementation. Magnesium deficiency occasionally causes hypocalcemia and hypophosphatemia. Hypophosphatemia usually results from the tremendous uptake of phosphate into cells during feeding. Hypophosphatemia can occur very rapidly, resulting in heart failure and death within days of feeding, the so-called "refeeding syndrome."

7.3 Refeeding syndrome

Definition

The term "refeeding syndrome" has two different meanings (Figure 7.4). The first is the non-specific symptoms that occur in patients who are renourished.

Table 7.7. *Nutritional deficiencies*

Deficiency	Store	Symptoms and signs	Features of deficiency	Monitoring and treatment	Length of treatment
Magnesium	Weeks to months	Muscle cramp Weakness (proximal myopathy) Fatigue of the focus of the eye Impaired short-term memory	While a low level always indicates deficiency, most deficiencies occur in the face of normal serum magnesium. A magnesium load test is required if the test is normal and symptoms of muscle cramping, muscle weakness, fatigue of the focus of the eye, or impaired memory are present	Preferred route is intravenous magnesium Magnesium can be given intramuscularly but is painful Oral magnesium is absorbed very poorly but can be used in addition to other routes or as prophylaxis	Usually requires five to ten intravenous treatments until symptoms disappear and serum levels remain normal. Gold standard of adequate repletion is magnesium load test at the end of treatment
Phosphorus	Days to weeks	Usually presents as the sudden onset of congestive heart failure	Independent of body stores Level drops immediately after eating and rises quickly with ingestion of phosphorus A falling or subnormal level is an indicator of increased risk of the medical consequences of phosphate deficiency (e.g. congestive heart failure, Wernicke–Korsakoff syndrome) and must be treated	Daily serum phosphorus during rapid weight gain (1 kg per week or more), then three times a week for three weeks, then once a week, if gaining 0.5 kg or more a week	Provide prophylaxis for as long as, and whenever, rapid weight gain occurs, plus for another two weeks Give at least 500 mg of phosphorus three times a day during the first week of refeeding and continue at this level if weight gain is 1.0 kg or more a week. More weight gain later drops to 0.5 kg a week or less, reduce rate to 500 mg of phosphorus once a day. Continue for as long as weight is gained at more than 0.5 kg a week

(cont.)

143

Table 7.7. (cont.)

Deficiency	Store	Symptoms and signs	Features of deficiency	Monitoring and treatment	Length of treatment
Potassium	Days to a week	Muscle weakness (proximal myopathy) Palpitations	Serum level is fairly proportional to total body stores. Serum potassium is elevated spuriously in acidemia and tissue injury (hemolysis in the blood tube will raise the level), and lowered with alkalosis. Serum potassium usually drops because of potassium loss in vomitus, but can drop because of lack of renal reabsorption due to magnesium deficiency. If the kidney is wasting more than 5 mm/l of potassium on a single urine sample, in the face of low serum potassium, suspect magnesium deficiency as the cause	Daily serum potassium for the first week of rapid weight gain, then three times a week for as long as weight gain continues at greater than 1 kg per week. Later, if weight gain continues at 0.5 kg a week, it need only be measured once a week	Provide prophylaxis of 24 mEq KCl two to three times a day. Increase the dose if there is a deficiency
Calcium	Months to years	Muscle cramping, carpopedal spasm (latent tetany), palpitations, dysrhythmias, seizures	Level of free (unbound) calcium in the blood is normally controlled carefully by serum parathormone. Low levels of serum calcium in AN indicate the protein that carries calcium is low but the free level is not low (measure serum free calcium – which will be normal) or there is a total body magnesium deficiency (causes low calcium by reducing the parathormone effect and secretion). The treatment of the latter is magnesium deficiency treatment	Measure serum calcium at the beginning of refeeding to rule out primary calcium abnormality. Do not repeat measurement unless muscle cramping or carpopedal spasm occurs	If ionized calcium is low, and cause is not total body magnesium deficiency, the treatment and treatment duration depend on the underlying cause

(cont.)

Table 7.7. (cont.)

Deficiency	Store	Symptoms and signs	Features of deficiency	Monitoring and treatment	Length of treatment
Thiamine	Days to weeks	Wernicke's encephalopathy (confusion, nystagmus or ophthalmoplegia, and ataxia) Much less commonly neuropathy or congestive heart failure	Deficiency can by precipitated by intravenous glucose	Avoid intravenous glucose. Monitor for and treat hypophosphatemia and hypomagnesemia. If Wernicke's is present, give thiamine 100 mg intravenously and intramuscularly immediately and 100 mg intramuscularly daily for ten days and correct hypophosphatemia and hypomagnesemia	Treat acute Wernicke's with 20 days of thiamine and correction of phosphorus and magnesium deficiencies
Iron	Months to years	Tiredness, pica (abnormal food cravings, the most common being for ice and cold beverages), anemia	Serum ferritin often low in AN due to very low oral intake	Supplementation can cause constipation, black stools, and upset stomach. Start supplementation with concurrent anemia or after initial refeeding is progressing well. Give ferrous sulfate, gluconate or fumarate 300 mg once a day, increasing gradually to three times a day if tolerated.	Iron supplementation should be continued for six months without anemia and for 12 months with associated anemia

(cont.)

145

Table 7.7. (cont.)

Deficiency	Store	Symptoms and signs	Features of deficiency	Monitoring and treatment	Length of treatment
Folic acid	Weeks	Tiredness, anemia	Serum folic acid changes quickly with diet, so red blood cell (RBC) folate should be ordered instead. RBC folate is usually normal in AN. If the RBC folate is low, this is usually due to decreased intake of green leafy vegetables. Folate is used quickly in cell production (particularly red blood cells), so it should be supplemented when iron or vitamin B12 is given for anemia, irrespective of its level. High RBC folate is usually due to ingestion of vitamin that contains folate	Folic acid orally 5 mg	Folic acid supplementation should be continued for a month, but longer if the hemoglobin is rising or if the diet is low in green, leafy vegetables
Vitamin B12	Three or five years	Tiredness and fatigue, yellowish skin and sclera, anemia, dementia, loss of normal gait and vibration and joint position sense, peripheral neuropathy	Vitamin B12 is only absorbed in the terminal ileum and only if bound to intrinsic factor produced in the stomach. It is stored in the liver and is necessary for cell division through the body. A low level is usually due to dietary deficiency, but about 3–9% of the time is due to malabsorption. Schilling's test is necessary to determine	Vitamin B12 by injection 1000 μg daily for three days and then 100 μg monthly for three to five years. If Schilling's test is normal, give the injections for six months and then use oral vitamin B12 tables 50 μg a day. Do not give tables with vitamin C or iron at the same time as	Continue for three to five years. If there is an abnormal Schilling's test, there may have to be lifelong supplementation. However, usually the abnormal Schilling's test is due to vitamin B12 or folate deficiency, causing intestinal cell atrophy, so the Schilling's test should be rechecked in a (cont.)

Table 7.7. (cont.)

Deficiency	Store	Symptoms and signs	Features of deficiency	Monitoring and treatment	Length of treatment
			whether malabsorption is the cause of B12 deficiency	vitamin B12 tablets because these decrease its absorption	few years and parenteral supplementation stopped
Vitamin K	One or more weeks	Delayed bleeding or bruising after trauma	The bacteria in the bowel manufacture vitamin K. The absorbed vitamin K is necessary for the production of all the coagulation factors except, factor VIII. Vitamin K deficiency is assessed indirectly by measurement of the coagulation by ordering an INR. Vitamin K deficiency causes a raised INR.	Treatment is by the injection of a solution of 10 mg of vitamin K, or if absorption is certain and there is no acute bleeding give 10 mg vitamin K orally for five days	One injection or five days of oral vitamin K
Anemia			A level of 10 g/l is to be expected in AN due to the "anemia of chronic disease" that is usually a secondary sideroblastic anemia that needs no treatment other than treatment of AN		
			A level lower than this may be due to iron deficiency, vitamin B12 deficiency, folate deficiency, self-phlebotomy, marrow failure, copper deficiency, or drug toxicity. A hematologist should inspect the blood film (RBC		

(cont.)

147

Table 7.7. (cont.)

Deficiency	Store	Symptoms and signs	Features of deficiency	Monitoring and treatment	Length of treatment
			morphology). Ferritin, vitamin B12, and RBC folate should be ordered with a hemoglobin of less than 10 g/l. Hematological consultation should be obtained if cause is not clear		
Vitamin A	17 years	Night blindness, Bitot's spots (appearance is like little bits of meringue on the sclera), collapse of globe of the eye	Measuring serum vitamin A levels can assess vitamin A deficiency. This test is expensive and should be ordered only if a deficiency is suspected. Vitamin A is bound in the blood to retinal binding globulin (RBG), which is synthesized in the liver. Patients who have severe protein deficiency (low albumen) or liver impairment may have a low serum vitamin A due to a low RBG level, with no deficiency of vitamin A. Conversely, when the RBG gets very low, vitamin A cannot be delivered to the tissues, even with treatment, and tissue damage due to vitamin A deficiency will occur	Treatment is oral vitamin A 5000–50 000 i.u. per day depending on the seriousness of the deficiency. If too much vitamin A is ingested, toxicity results, leading to many systemic symptoms, including bone aches and symptoms resulting from increased intracranial pressure	Continue vitamin A for a few months. During that time, assess and increase vitamin A in diet if possible, and start a multivitamin that contains vitamin A
Pyridoxine	Months to years	Peripheral neuro-pathy, anemia	Deficiency is rare in AN	Treat deficiency with 100 mg pyridoxine per day	Continue oral pyridoxine for three months

(cont.)

Table 7.7. (cont.)

Deficiency	Store	Symptoms and signs	Features of deficiency	Monitoring and treatment	Length of treatment
Zinc	Weeks to months	Weight loss, impaired or abnormal taste (dysgeusia), dry and peeling skin (especially on palms and soles), decreased cellular immune function	Zinc is found mainly in milk products and seafood and is bound to fiber in the diet. Copper and zinc compete for the same absorptive pathway. If copper is taken in large quantities for long periods of time, zinc deficiency may develop, and vice versa. Zinc intake in AN, especially with quasi-vegetarian diets, is very low. Estrogen increases urine loss of zinc. In AN, zinc deficiency usually presents as dry skin and decreased taste sensation. Serum zinc can be measured but does not reflect zinc stores unless it is low. Zinc is bound to albumen and zinc-binding globulin, so patients with low serum protein will appear to have low serum zinc despite normal free serum zinc. Zinc deficiency can be measured by taste testing (e.g. the Accusens t-test), but we have not found this sensitive or specific to zinc deficiency	Give 14–28 mg a day of elemental zinc (zinc gluconate 100–200 mg per day) for two months	Routine treatment with zinc in AN for two months. Treat deficiency state for six months

149

(cont.)

Table 7.7. (cont.)

Deficiency	Store	Symptoms and signs	Features of deficiency	Monitoring and treatment	Length of treatment
Riboflavin		Angular stomatitis		Prevent by giving a daily multivitamin. Treatment of the deficiency is with a multi B vitamin for one month	One month and then multivitamin for a year
Copper		Megaloblastic anemia, thrombocytopenia, leukopenia, together or individually	Copper deficiency is rare in AN. The bone marrow shows changes indistinguishable from those seen in folate or vitamin B12 deficiency. Suspect copper deficiency with anemia, thrombocytopenia, or leukopenia that is progressive and undiagnosed and appears megaloblastic. Taking 400 mg or more of zinc gluconate a day for more than four months can cause copper deficiency	Treat with a few milligrams a day of oral elemental copper as the sulfate form	Three months

(cont.)

Table 7.7. (cont.)

Deficiency	Store	Symptoms and signs	Features of deficiency	Monitoring and treatment	Length of treatment
Selenium	17-year store	Proximal myopathy, cardiomyopathy	Found in fruits and vegetables. It is low in the soil in New Zealand, parts of Canada, and China. Marketed vegetables come from around the world, so low selenium ingestion is rare. Selenium is necessary for the metabolic function of mitochondria. A deficiency is usually caused by malabsorption coupled with low intake. Deficiency is very rare in AN. Suspect selenium deficiency if a severe undiagnosed myopathy develops in a patient with chronic severe AN. Low serum level is not diagnostic of a clinical deficiency	Treat symptomatic deficiency with intravenous selenium, as administered to patients receiving total parenteral nutrition. Treat low serum level with oral vitamin containing selenium	

Clinical meaning   **Nutritional meaning**

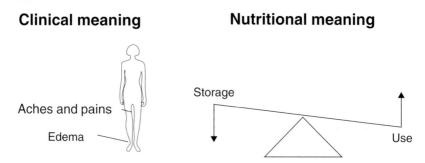

Aches and pains

Edema

Figure 7.4. The two meanings of the term "refeeding syndrome".

These consist of dependent edema and aches and pains, especially in the legs. The dependent edema, often referred to as "refeeding edema," occurs even if the patient has a normal fluid volume and albumen level. It is due to the impaired renal function and low metabolic rate present at the beginning of feeding. The edema is much greater if there is pretreatment volume depletion and low albumen.

The second meaning of the term is the complex of deficiencies that can develop as a consequence of feeding. The following sections explain this potentially lethal consequence of feeding and how to prevent and treat it. Table 7.8 presents a protocol to prevent the refeeding syndrome.

Why does the refeeding syndrome occur?

The refeeding syndrome is best understood by analogy. Imagine the building site of a skyscraper just as the first floor is completed. The site would be covered with all manner of building materials, including steel, wood, nails, and glass. It would seem that there should be plenty of materials to continue building. However, we know that the materials are likely to run out after a few floors. Even more importantly, some materials will run out much sooner than others. So it is with refeeding. The malnourished body has, at the beginning of refeeding, inadequate nutrients to continue the process of rebuilding the body for long. Also, the amount of each nutrient that is stored in the body is highly variable. Typically, stores of vitamin K last a couple of weeks, those of vitamin B12 last a few years, and those of selenium last a couple of decades. AN is also associated with bizarre eating habits, e.g. patients may ingest only watermelon or oranges for months. Feeding delivers carbohydrate and some fat and protein, but only modest amounts of vitamins and minerals. This explains why the initial blood work is usually normal in AN, and why a variety of deficiencies develop during refeeding.

Table 7.8. *Suggested protocol to prevent refeeding syndrome*

Dietician to order diet (start with low-calorie diet and increase gradually)
Laboratory:

- hemoglobin, white blood cell count, platelet estimation, serum sodium, potassium, chloride, bicarbonate, blood urea nitrogen, creatinine, aspartate transaminase, alkaline phosphatase, magnesium, calcium, phosphorus, ferritin, vitamin B12, red blood cell folate, zinc, international normalized ratio (INR)
- electrocardiogram
- Urinalysis, routine and microscopy

Routine blood work: potassium, phosphorus, and magnesium daily for seven days and then every Monday, Wednesday, and Friday

Routine supplements:

- potassium chloride (pills, effervescent, or liquid) 24 mEq three times a day for 21 days
- sodium phosphate solution 5 ml (550 mg of phosphorus) three times a day for 21 days
- multivitamins two tablets a day for two months and then one tablet a day
- thiamine 100 mg a day for five days
- zinc gluconate 100 mg daily for two months.

Note: oral magnesium is not absorbed adequately. Oral magnesium may be enough to prevent serum magnesium levels dropping, masking a significant total body deficiency. Therefore, monitor serum magnesium and treat with parenteral magnesium.

Intravenous rehydration if required: give normal saline (0.9% NaCl solution) at 100–150 cm^3 per hour until intravascular volume is normalized.

The symptoms that occur during refeeding are those of the specific deficiencies that develop. The deficiencies that can cause death – potassium, magnesium, and phosphate – must be monitored and prevented.

7.4 Nutrition in eating disorders

Macronutrients

There are no essential carbohydrates. Linoleic acid is likely the only essential fatty acid in humans; it is required in only very small amounts. The amino acids are the building blocks of proteins. Proteins cannot be made without amino acids and energy. There are a number of essential amino acids. Carbohydrate and protein have 4 kcal per gram; fat has 9 kcal per gram.

Energy

Energy comes from the ingested macronutrients (fat, carbohydrate, protein). Energy malnutrition is always present in AN. With malnutrition, energy stores are used in the following order: carbohydrate stores, fat stores, protein stores.

Tip for feeding: a combination of carbohydrates, fats, and proteins should be used.

Protein

The protein intake and the protein mass are usually very low in AN. The quality of the essential amino acids in different foods varies.

Tip for feeding: between 0.7 and 1.5 g of protein per kilogram of body weight in a variety of food sources should be used.

Fat

Essential fatty acid deficiency has not been reported in AN. Most patients with AN, however, ingest very little fat. Malnutrition causes elevated serum cholesterol in AN due to reduced clearance by the liver. The treatment for this is feeding, not a lipid-lowering medication or a reduction of dietary fat.

Tip for feeding: compared with protein and carbohydrates, fat has more than twice the number of calories per gram and is less filling. It is an essential part of feeding.

Fat-soluble vitamins

The fat-soluble vitamins are K, A, D, and E.

Vitamin K

This is manufactured by bacteria in the bowel. The absorbed vitamin K is necessary for the production of a number of coagulation factors (II, VII, IX, X). Deficiency causes delayed clotting and bruising. Vitamin K deficiency is assessed indirectly by measurement of the coagulation by ordering an international normalized ratio (INR). Vitamin K deficiency causes a raised INR. Treatment is by injection of a solution of 10 mg of vitamin K.

Vitamin A

The body usually has a 17-year store of vitamin A. Vitamin A deficiency causes night blindness, followed by changes in the globe of the eye (Bitot's spots, which look like little bits of meringue on the white of the eye) and then collapse of the eyeball. Measuring serum vitamin A levels can assess vitamin A deficiency. This test is expensive and should be ordered only if a deficiency is suspected.

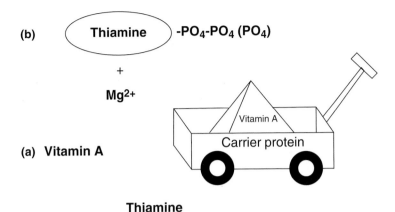

Figure 7.5. (a) Vitamin A requires a specialized protein to reach the tissues. (b) Thiamine requires magnesium and phosphorus to function.

Vitamin A is bound in the blood to retinal binding globulin (RBG), which is made in the liver (Figure 7.5a). Patients with severe protein deficiency (low albumen) or liver impairment may have a low serum vitamin A due to a low RBG level, with no vitamin A deficiency. However, if the RBG gets very low, then vitamin A cannot be delivered to the tissues, even with supplementation, and the tissue damage due to vitamin A deficiency will occur.

Treatment is with oral vitamin A, 5000–50 000 IU per day, depending on the seriousness of the deficiency. If too much vitamin A is ingested, toxicity causes bone aches and increased intracranial pressure.

Vitamin D

Vitamin D is obtained in food and by exposure of the skin to sunlight. It is metabolized to its active form by the kidney. Deficiency causes abnormal calcium homeostasis, leading to low serum calcium, osteomalacia, muscle weakness, tetany, and seizures. Vitamin D can be administered orally in a multivitamin in a dose of 400 IU per day. An excess of vitamin D will cause hypercalcemia, which results in polyuria, polydipsia, volume depletion, confusion, and chemosis (red sclera).

Vitamin E

A deficiency in vitamin E may cause vascular abnormalities. There is no report of vitamin E deficiency in AN.

The water-soluble vitamins

Folic acid

Folic acid (folate) is present in the diet mainly in green, leafy vegetables (derived from the Latin *folia*, meaning leaf). Folate is necessary for protein formation. Folic acid deficiency will result in a megalobastic anemia, confusion, and tiredness. The store of folate in the body is not great. Thus, during refeeding, folic acid deficiency may occur. Measure the serum red blood cell (RBC) folate rather than the serum folate, because serum folate does not reflect body folic acid stores as well. Treatment is 5 mg of folic acid a day by tablet.

Thiamine (vitamin B1)

Thiamine is required in the amount of about 1 mg per day. Both beriberi and Wernicke–Korsakoff syndrome result from thiamine deficiency. Wernicke–Korsakoff syndrome is the combination of Wernicke's encephalopathy, the acute result of thiamine deficiency in the brain, and Korsakoff syndrome, the long-term result of thiamine deficiency in the brain. Wernicke–Korsakoff syndrome is seen with deficiency of phosphate or magnesium, because they are necessary for the function of thiamine (Figure 7.5b). Wernicke's encephalopathy can be precipitated by the administration of intravenous glucose. The rapid elevation of glucose uses up the remaining thiamine and precipitates the deficiency. Wernicke's encephalopathy is due to cellular dysfunction of the brain cells around the third and fourth ventricles, the mammillary bodies, and the aqueduct. When the dysfunction begins, there is confusion, ataxia, and nystagmus or ophthalmoplegia. Over the space of hours to a day, the affected cells die and the signs gradually settle into a permanent short-term memory deficit. This may or may not be associated with confabulation (insertion of fancied memories for those not remembered, the fancied memories lasting for the duration of short-term recall, which is usually about one hour). Wet beriberi causes congestive heart failure due to a weakened dilated heart; dry beriberi causes peripheral neuropathy. Neither type of beriberi has been reported in AN.

When refeeding begins, administer thiamine 100 mg orally for five days. Avoid intravenous glucose. Monitor for and treat hypophosphatemia and hypomagnesemia. If Wernicke's is present, give thiamine 100 mg intravenously and intramuscularly immediately, and then 100 mg intramuscularly for ten days, and correct hypophosphatemia and hypomagnesemia.

Riboflavin

Riboflavin is a water-soluble B vitamin present in small quantities in food. A deficiency causes angular stomatitis. Prevent deficiency by giving a daily multivitamin. Treatment of deficiency is with a multi-B vitamin for one month.

Niacin

Niacin is a water-soluble B vitamin present in small quantities in food. Deficiency causes pellagra. Pellagra can cause the "4 Ds:" diarrhea, dermatitis, dementia, and death. The only characteristic sign of pellagra is the flaky, hyperpigmented rash seen on the anterior shin (see Section 4.3). Prevent by giving a multivitamin once daily. Niacin can cause flushing, itching, and dizziness. The flushing and itching can be prevented by taking 80 mg of acetylsalicylic acid per day, or by increasing the dose more gradually.

Pyridoxine (vitamin B6)

Pyridoxine is a water-soluble B vitamin. Deficiency causes peripheral neuropathy and sideroblastic anemia. Deficiency is rare in AN. Prevent by giving a multivitamin daily. Treat deficiency with 100 mg pyridoxine a day for a few months.

Cyanocobalamin (vitamin B12)

Vitamin B12 is a water-soluble vitamin that is low in vegetarian diets. It is necessary for cell division. Deficiency results in megaloblastic anemia, organic brain syndrome, subacute combined degeneration of the cord (a combination of upper motor neuron weakness from involvement of the extrapyramidal tract and loss of proprioception and joint position sense from involvement of the posterior columns), peripheral neuropathy, tiredness, jaundice (due to ineffective erythropoesis), and congestive cardiomyopathy.

Vitamin B12 deficiency is usually due to decreased intake during a time of growth, when requirements are high. About 3% of cases of vitamin B12 deficiency in AN are due to impaired absorption as a result of pernicious anemia (an autoimmune disorder that causes decreased intrinsic factor production from the stomach due to antibodies against the parietal cells, where it is formed) or disease such as Crohn's or celiac disease, which cause decreased absorption in the terminal ileum, the only part of the bowel where the vitamin B12–instrinsic factor complex can be absorbed.

A Schilling's test should be performed to rule out B12 malabsorption. Then give vitamin B12 1000 μg a day for three days, followed by three years of either 100 μg intramuscularly a month or 50 μg a day orally if absorption is normal and the patient can be relied upon to eat and not purge. The absorption of oral vitamin B12 is decreased by concomitant ingestion of vitamin C or iron.

Biotin

Deficiency of biotin is very rare and occurs only with the ingestion of raw egg whites. Raw egg whites contain avidin, which binds biotin, preventing its absorption. Biotin deficiency causes skin exfoliation. Prevention is by avoiding raw egg whites in the diet. If deficiency is present, then biotin should be given and raw egg white ingestion stopped.

Minerals

Potassium

Potassium is a mineral (cation), most of which resides inside the cell. It is present in the diet in large amounts in potatoes, oranges, and bananas. Deficiency occurs with vomiting, diarrhea, diuretics, and rapid refeeding. The symptoms of deficiency are weakness, tiredness, and palpitations. The signs of deficiency are a proximal myopathy and dysrhythmias.

For treatment, oral potassium of any variety (pills, liquid, effervescent tablets) or intravenous 20–40 mEq of potassium chloride per liter of normal saline at 75–150 cm^3/hour (if the patient is not passing urine due to renal dysfunction, then death from hyperkalemia may result). Use the intravenous route if the patient cannot take oral potassium, if the potassium continues to fall despite oral potassium, or if the potassium is less than 2.5 mEq/l.

Calcium

Calcium is a mineral (cation) that resides almost entirely inside bone and cells. The bones hold a large store of calcium, so low intake of calcium is not a cause of hypocalcemia in AN. Low serum calcium is due to either a low carrier protein (with normal ionized calcium and therefore no disturbance of calcium homeostasis) or difficulty with the regulation of calcium homeostasis. The latter cause is usually due to total body magnesium deficiency in AN. Magnesium deficiency decreases the amount of calcium absorbed, the amount of calcium retained by the kidney, the amount of parathormone secreted, the effect that parathormone has on bone, and the release of calcium from bone independent of the effect of parathormone. Eighty percent of patients with magnesium deficiency will develop low serum calcium over time.

Measure the ionized calcium or estimate the amount of binding protein in the blood by measuring albumen. Suspect magnesium deficiency if the ionized calcium is low. If neither is the cause, then rule out other causes, including renal failure, total abstinence from sunlight, and hypoparathyroidism.

Magnesium

Magnesium is a mineral (cation) that resides almost entirely (99%) within cells. About 50% of intracellular magnesium is in bones and muscles. Magnesium is present in small amounts in the diet. About 4–6 mmol of magnesium is absorbed per day. Magnesium is absorbed poorly and has laxative properties (milk of magnesium, magnesium-containing antacids, magnesium citrate, etc.). All of the magnesium that is absorbed is normally excreted to maintain magnesium homeostasis in the body. Magnesium is necessary for many of the metabolic pathways in the body. Deficiency causes proximal myopathy, muscle cramping (especially at night and in the large muscles of the legs), impaired short-term memory, and difficulty in maintaining visual focus on near objects for more than half an hour. Serum magnesium is not a good indicator of total body magnesium. Low serum magnesium is always associated with low total body magnesium; most patients with low total body magnesium have normal serum magnesium, however. During magnesium treatment, the serum magnesium may even be high, despite low total body magnesium.

Tables 7.9 and 7.10 summarize the treatment of magnesium deficiency. Treat all patients with low serum magnesium, and screen those with normal serum magnesium for deficiency with the magnesium load test. The load test consists of administering 20 mmol magnesium sulfate intravenously in 250 cm^3 normal saline for four hours, with a 24-hour urine collection for magnesium that begins after voiding, just before the infusion is begun. Normally, all of the administered magnesium is excreted in the urine. If the patient puts out less than 15 mmol of magnesium, they are deficient.

Caution: do not give magnesium to patients who are not voiding urine (renal failure). Severe hypermagnesemia causes death due to heart failure. This occurs at about three times the upper limit of serum magnesium and is preceded by a loss of deep tendon reflexes.

Phosphorus/phosphate

Phosphorus is a mineral (anion) that is primarily intracellular. It is present in many foods, especially milk-based products. It is absorbed rapidly and easily, moves into the blood quickly, moves into cells with glucose with a corresponding drop in blood phosphorus after meals, and is lost rapidly in the urine with any diuresis. Phosphorus is part of ATP, cAMP, and 2,3-DPG and is therefore essential to the moment-to-moment functioning of the body. Hypophosphatemia results in every organ in the body rapidly losing function, followed by cell death and lysis. The earliest sign is heart failure.

Hypophosphatemia must be prevented. All patients during refeeding must be given oral phosphate, in a dose of at least 500 mg twice a day. This can be given as a tablet or, much less expensively, as phosphate solution (a very large dose has laxative properties, whereas a dose or 5 ml or 550 mg two or three times a day does not cause diarrhea). A phosphate level that is dropping (even within

Table 7.9. *Options for magnesium supplementation*

Route	Medications	Orders	Benefits and limitations
Oral	Magnesium glucoheptonate (magnesium rougier) 5 ml three times a day Magnesium gluconate one tablet three times a day Calcium–magnesium oral tablets, one tablet three times a day	Three times a day for weeks to months	Very little is absorbed. The oral route should not be used to treat symptomatic deficiencies, but it can be used as an adjunctive therapy or to prevent deficiency. Taking too much will cause diarrhea
Intramuscular	10 cm^3 vial of magnesium sulfate 50% solution contains 20 mmol magnesium, 40 mEq of magnesium, and 5 g of magnesium sulfate	2 cm^3 intramuscularly in one or both buttocks For the treatment of symptomatic deficiency, give one injection hourly for six hours, then one injection every four hours for five days	Fast, inexpensive Amount incorporated into cells is more than with intravenous because it is absorbed from the intramuscular route more slowly However, injections often cause pain, and many injections are required because only 2 cm^3 can be given intramuscularly
Intravenous	Same as intramuscular solution	20 mmol of magnesium sulfate in 250 cm^3 of 0.9% saline over four hours daily for five to ten days	Raises the serum and tissue levels quickly, resulting in symptomatic improvement However, need for daily intravenous infusions limits availability of treatment Note: overdosing and underdosing are common because 40 mEq of magnesium = 20 mmol of magnesium = 10 cm^3 of 50% solution = 5 g of magnesium sulfate *Use SI units only*

Table 7.10. *Performing and interpreting magnesium load test*

Instruct the patient to empty their bladder before the infusion begins.

Begin a urine collection for 24 hours to measure magnesium, volume, and total creatinine.

Start intravenous solution of magnesium sulfate 20 mmol (10 cm^3 of 50% solution of magnesium sulfate) in 250 cm^3 of 0.9% saline to be given with a volume regulator (so it does not run in quickly) over four hours.

Discontinue intravenous (or cap the saline lock).

Nursing instructions:

- The patient must remain recumbent for the first 30 minutes of the infusion.
- Observe for hypotension, flushing, and intestinal cramps at the beginning of the infusion.
- Instruct the patient to continue to collect their urine for 24 hours and to bring the collection back to the laboratory for analysis.

In normal humans, the kidney clears all of the magnesium administered intravenously within 24 hours. Patients who are deficient put out 15 mmol or less.

Important: magnesium must not be administered in renal failure. Magnesium is excreted only by the kidney, and very high serum magnesium can cause heart failure.

the normal range) must be treated by increasing oral phosphate. A phosphate level that is dropping quickly, or is less than half the normal level, must be treated by discontinuing all refeeding and administering oral and intravenous phosphate. Intravenous phosphate is given as a potassium phosphate mixture – request directions from your pharmacist.

Zinc

Zinc is a mineral (cation) that is found primarily in cells. It is an important part of many enzymatic processes. Zinc deficiency causes weight loss, impaired or abnormal taste (dysgeusia), dry and peeling skin (especially on the palms and soles), and decreased cellular immune function. Zinc is found mainly in milk products and seafoods and is bound to fiber in the diet. Copper and zinc compete for the same absorptive pathway; if copper is taken in large quantities for long periods of time, then zinc deficiency may develop, and vice versa. Zinc intake is low in AN, especially in patients following quasi-vegetarian diets. Estrogen increases urine loss of zinc. Serum zinc can be measured but does not reflect zinc stores unless it is low. Zinc is bound to albumen and zinc-binding globulin; low serum protein will cause low serum zinc, although free serum zinc may be normal. Zinc deficiency can be measured by taste testing (e.g. the

Accusens t-test); however, we have not found this to be sensitive or specific to zinc deficiency. The one double-blinded, randomized, controlled trial of zinc in AN demonstrated doubling of the rate of increase in BMI in patients treated with oral zinc, independent of the serum zinc level.

All patients should be treated with 14–28 mg a day of elemental zinc (zinc gluconate 100 mg/day) for two months. If serum zinc is low, or if symptoms of zinc deficiency exist (acrodermatitis, dysgeusia), then continue the treatment for six months or until the intake of zinc is normal.

Selenium

The body has a 17-year store of this trace mineral (cation). Selenium is found in fruits and vegetables, but it is low in the soil in New Zealand, parts of Canada, and China. A low intake of selenium is rare because marketed vegetables come from various locations. Selenium is necessary for the metabolic function of mitochondria. Deficiency is usually caused by a combination of low intake and malabsorption. Selenium deficiency in AN is very rare. It presents with proximal myopathy, cardiomyopathy (Keshan disease), and liver dysfunction. Suspect selenium deficiency if a severe undiagnosed myopathy develops in a patient with chronic severe AN. Prevent selenium deficiency by giving a multivitamin containing a small amount of selenium. Treatment involves intravenous selenium, as administered to patients receiving total parenteral nutrition.

Copper

Copper is a trace element that acts as a coenzyme. Copper deficiency is rare in AN. It presents as a megaloblastic anemia, thrombocytopenia, and leukopenia, together or individually. The bone marrow shows changes indistinguishable from those seen in folate or vitamin B12 deficiency. Suspect copper deficiency with an undiagnosed megaloblastic anemia, thrombocytopenia, or leukopenia. Ingesting at least 400 mg of zinc gluconate a day for four months can cause deficiency of copper. Prevent deficiency by ingestion of a multivitamin containing a few milligrams of copper per day.

7.5 Guidelines for refeeding

Methods of refeeding

Feeding can be done orally, by nasogastric tube, by parenteral nutrition, or by gastrostomy.

The oral route is always preferred because it has the fewest potential complications and it will be the route of feeding on discharge.

The nasogastric route is the second best route for feeding. It employs the gut, which encourages return of normal gastrointestinal function and regulates absorption. The nasogastric tube can be uncomfortable, both when inserted and afterwards. However, if the tube is inserted medially and slightly downward in the most patent nares, and if the tube is then advanced at the rate of esophageal peristalsis while having the patient swallow (sitting upright, head slightly forward, sucking water through a straw), discomfort is minimized. A silastic tube should be used because it softens to the consistency of the body after being inserted. The shorter (stomach-length) tube rather than the longer (duodenal-length) tube should be used because the longer tube has a much larger tip. Gel can be put on the end of the tube to lubricate the nares for insertion. If the patient is very sensitive to discomfort, then lidocaine gel should be used. The lidocaine takes time to work, so it must be inserted into the nares minutes before the insertion. Sublingual lorazepam 1 or 2 mg a few minutes before the insertion may also be needed if anxiety is severe. The position of the tube should be checked by X-ray to ensure that it is in the stomach and not the lung.

Many patients will covertly withdraw the tube to purge, only to reinsert it afterwards. An X-ray should be repeated to check the positioning if this has happened. Do not use nasal clips to secure the tube, as they are not esthetically acceptable. Use non-allergic tape to secure the tube, which should be draped gently over the ipsilateral ear.

The tube can be left in situ for up to six weeks, but it will usually block sooner with intermittent feeding. To prevent blockage, grind up one or two pancreatic enzyme tablets in sterile fluid and insert the mixture into the tube every few days. This mixture can also be used to unblock a clogged tube. Do not use acid or force to unblock the tube. Acid may react with the tube, while force can perforate the stomach.

Either gravity drip or a feeding pump can be used to regulate the rate of feeding. Pumps must incorporate a device that shuts off feeding should the resistance continue to increase.

Feedings may be given constantly, intermittently, for part of the day, or as a combination. The important points are to make sure that you are not feeding when the patient has the best chance of tampering and that a gastric residual does not build up over about 400 cm^3.

Parenteral nutrition

Parenteral nutrition should be used in eating disorders only when a period of nutrition is absolutely needed that cannot be achieved in any other way. This might be the case with superior mesenteric artery syndrome, for example. Parenteral nutrition introduces the potential complications of venous clot, infection, pneumothorax, and fluid overload. Also, the patient may fiddle with the tubing: the authors have had patients disconnect the tubing and drain the feeding fluids, which could cause air embolism and death.

Gastrostomy

Gastrostomy tubes allow feeding, like nasogastric feeding, but with a reduced risk of reflux. It also reduces the chance of the patient tampering with the feeding tube, although this is still possible.

Rate and frequency of increasing feeding

Deficiencies should be corrected before feeding. Then, feeding may be begun with 600–800 calories per day, increasing gradually every four to seven days until the rate of weight gain is 1 kg a week. The number of calories required for feeding is highly variable: as little as 1400 calories a day or as much as 4500 calories a day may be required. Most patients, however, will require about 2400 calories a day. High levels of anxiety, exercise, cigarette smoking, and purging all increase the calorie requirement.

Supplement formulas usually have one calorie per gram, so 300 ml will therefore have 300 calories. Other formulas have 1.5 or two calories per milliliter. The likelihood of the feeding tube becoming clogged is increased with more viscous feeds (higher concentration of calories). Some formulas are milk (lactose)-based; these will cause diarrhea in lactase-deficient (milk intolerance) patients.

Meal support

Meal support is the single most important advance in the feeding of severely ill patients with AN and BN. Meal support means a planned staff meal intervention designed to reduce stress and increase success with eating.

A dietitian plans the meals. Meal slips come up with the meals so that the meal support staff are aware of the planned intake. Rules are reviewed with patients and staff regarding meals. For example, no diet foods may be consumed, only a few specific replacement foods are allowed and only under certain circumstances, food cannot be tampered with (e.g. dabbed, mixed, overheated), patients must remain at the table during meals and for a total of 45 minutes – even if they have finished their meal – and discussion must not revolve around eating, weight, or portion size.

Meals are eaten together, although a separate table for patients who are capable of taking more responsibility is preferable. The milieu, including the setting, conversation, and music, must be conducive to relieving stress.

Meal support can be done by any trained health care professional. As it can be very stressful, it is important to have as many staff share in the meal support as possible.

Warming

Hypothermia, increased sympathetic function, autonomic lability, abnormal intestinal peristalsis, parotid hypertrophy, and anxiety are common in AN. William Gull suggested warming as a treatment for AN in his initial description. Many patients drink warm liquids or expose themselves to heat, causing the permanent discoloration of erythema ab igne. With this in mind, the authors conducted a randomized, controlled trial of warming during meals. This has proved highly beneficial. Patients report feeling less full and more relaxed, and we have observed a more rapid reduction in the size of the parotid gland. It is possible that all of these findings are related to a reduction in sympathetic tone and an increase in parasympathetic tone, caused by warming. Parotid secretion is under the control of the autonomic nervous system. Our patients prefer wearing warming jackets routinely with eating.

7.6 Common nutritional problems

Problem 1: hypomagnesemia

Case

An 18-year-old female with AN complains of muscle cramps after seven days of feeding in hospital. On questioning, she has cramps of the muscles in her legs, especially at night, her short-term memory is impaired, and she can read books for only half an hour before she has to "strain her eyes" to read. Her serum magnesium is 0.7 mmol/l, which is the lower limit of normal. Over the seven days, her levels have dropped gradually from 0.9 mmol/l. A magnesium load test is administered. She is given 20 mmol magnesium sulfate in 250 ml of normal saline over four hours, and her urine is collected (after voiding) from the beginning of the infusion for 24 hours. She reports feeling much improved during the infusion and for one day after. The urine collection shows 15 mmol of magnesium, demonstrating that she retained some magnesium and was deficient. She is given a further ten daily infusions. A urine collection with the last infusion contained 20 mmol of magnesium.

Comment

Serum magnesium falls over five to ten days of feeding, resulting in symptoms of weakness, leg cramps at night, short-term memory impairment, and loss of visual focus after about 30 minutes. The latter is due to weakness of the ciliary muscles and resultant loss of adjustment of the shape of the lens. Regarding supplementation, oral magnesium results in diarrhea. In fact, many laxatives are magnesium salts – such as magnesium-containing antacids, milk of magnesium, and magnesium citrate. Intramuscular magnesium often, but not always, causes pain. Some patients prefer intramuscular injections of 2 cm^3 of 50% magnesium sulfate for supplementation due to its convenience in comparison to intravenous magnesium. Overall, it is best to give magnesium intravenously. Give 20 mmol in 250 cm^3 normal saline over four hours daily. Usually five to ten days of treatment is required. Comparing the dose given with the amount lost in the urine tests for sufficient administration. The urine should be collected for 24 hours from the beginning of the infusion. It is easy to give the wrong amount of magnesium because 10 cm^3 of 50% magnesium sulfate contains 5 g = 40 meq = 20 mmol. Always order in millimoles, as this is the SI unit that is used for measurement by the laboratory.

Nursing implications

- Magnesium deficiency may be present even with a normal serum magnesium.
- Magnesium supplementation is dangerous with renal failure because magnesium must be cleared through the urine.
- Magnesium infusion must be given over four hours or longer. A bolus of magnesium will cause death by stopping the heart.
- When magnesium is being delivered intravenously, it can cause some increase in urination, mild headache, bowel movements, and some lightheadedness due to vasodilation. Reassure the patient that this is normal.
- Once open, a vial of magnesium sulfate cannot be stored or reused. Magnesium will bind other medications, so do not mix medications with magnesium, and give intravenous magnesium by itself.
- Intramuscular magnesium hurts – but not severely. However, it is irritative and if given into a nerve will cause injury to that nerve.

Problem 2: hypophosphatemia

Case

A 17-year-old female with AN binge–purge subtype is admitted for feeding to the medical ward of a general hospital. Five days into feeding, she becomes short of breath and orthopneic. She is noticed to be tachycardic. On review, her serum phosphorus is 0.3 mmol/l (very low) and she is in congestive heart failure, with rales in her chest and increased jugular venous pressure. She is transferred to the intensive care unit.

Feeding is stopped. The patient is given intravenous and oral phosphorus for two days until her serum levels stabilize. She is transferred to the ward and feeding is recommenced. Once again, her serum phosphorus falls.

Comment

Phosphorus usually falls over the first few days, although it may fall much later. Usually, a fall in the serum level causes no symptoms. Symptoms usually begin at between one-third and one-half the lower normal laboratory limit. Importantly, the level will fall rapidly once the level is below normal. It is therefore essential to supplement routinely with 5 cm^3 of phosphate solution three times a day. If the level is low and dropping, then use oral and intravenous phosphorus and stop feeding. The first symptom of low phosphorus in AN is usually shortness of breath due to congestive heart failure, secondary to congestive cardiomyopathy. However, every cell in the body will fail (all cells need ATP), resulting in multisystem failure and death if not corrected.

Nursing implications

- There is usually no warning of congestive heart failure due to hypophosphatemia in AN, other than the decreasing serum levels.
- Oral phosphate can be given as pills or as 5 cm^3 of liquid. They both contain about 500 mg of phosphorus. If too much oral phosphate is taken, it will cause diarrhea because it is an osmotic agent.

Problem 3: hypokalemia

Case

A 27-year-old female bulimic presents to the office with weakness. Laboratory tests show potassium of 2.5 mmol/l. You prescribe oral potassium in increasing amounts, but the potassium does not correct. You examine the patient and find volume depletion (dehydration). You arrange intravenous saline to expand the volume, because the patient may be wasting potassium in the urine in order to retain sodium. The patient feels better, but her potassium is still low, and a urine sample shows that she is wasting potassium in the urine. A magnesium load test shows she is magnesium-deficient. Once you replete her magnesium, her potassium corrects with supplementation.

Comment

Potassium levels usually fall gradually. There are usually no symptoms. When symptoms do occur, they are weakness, palpitations, and polyuria. Give potassium orally or intravenously. If the levels are low, remember to exclude volume depletion, with renal exchange for sodium. Also, high urine potassium in a euvolemic patient often indicates magnesium depletion, as this causes the kidney to be unable to reabsorb potassium. There should be almost no potassium in the urine of a hypokalemic patient.

Nursing implications

Urine collection for potassium concentration is a spot sample, not a 24-hour collection.

Problem 4: Wernicke's encephalopathy

Case

A 24-year-old male anorexic presents to the outpatient clinic with dizziness and mild confusion. On examination, he has lateral nystagmus and perhaps a mild change in gait, and there is a collateral history of significant memory impairment over the past day. You test serum magnesium and phosphorus and administer 100 mg of thiamine intramuscularly and orally. Serum magnesium and phosphorus levels return as normal.

Thiamine deficiency may occur at any time, even early in feeding. Thiamine can be given orally, intramuscularly, or intravenously. It is adequate to give it orally unless a glucose load is to be given or a deficiency is suspected. In this case, give 100 mg both intramuscularly and intravenously. Thiamine is a water-soluble vitamin, so the intravenous dose will not linger long.

Nursing implications

- Sudden onset of difficulty with gait, double vision, or confusion is often due to medication side effects, but it can be due to Wernicke's encephalopathy.
- Thiamine must be given parenterally if the diagnosis of Wernicke's encephalopathy is made.

Problem 5: hypoglycemia

Case

You are asked to review a 27-year-old female with AN who has been admitted to the medical ward for feeding. She has been in hospital a few days and has been resistant and manipulative. The nurse says that she just lies in her bed and will not eat. On questioning, you consider a decreased level of consciousness rather than acting out and ask the nurse to take a blood sugar at the bedside immediately. She returns to the telephone to report a blood sugar of 1.9 mmol/l. The patient awakens after 50 ml of 50% dextrose is administered as a push intravenously. She is kept on 10% dextrose in water for several weeks. When the dextrose is reduced, she becomes hypoglycemic after meals and she continues to fail a glucagon test.

Comment

Hypoglycemia usually occurs when feeding is begun after recent low calorie intake. This is counterintuitive to many, who expect that it is more likely to occur before feeding begins. It is caused by the secretion of insulin in response to food, resulting in a drop in blood sugar that cannot be compensated for by the release of glucagon because of a lack of liver glycogen. In other words, the hypoglycemia develops in response to an increase in the release of insulin caused by the feeding. In normal people, the drop in blood sugar caused by the insulin would be corrected by the release of glucagon from the pancreas, which would release sugar from the liver. In early feeding, there is no glycogen to be broken down.

Use of the glucagon test

The glucagon test can be used to see whether the liver can release sugar to compensate for drops in blood sugar. Intravenous administration of 1 mg of glucagon in a fasting patient should result in the elevation of blood sugar to normal (a rise to above 7 mmol/l is normal). Measure fasting, 10-minute, and 20-minute blood sugars. We normally carry out the test once a week before breakfast. Patients will request that the test be done frequently because they do not like receiving dextrose intravenously. However, the treatment must not be terminated early because hypoglycemia usually takes one to two weeks to normalize and, if stopped prematurely, can lead to death.

Nursing implications

- Ensure that an intravenous line with normal saline is running before the test.
- The solution of glucagon requires the vial of fluid to be injected into the bottle of glucagon powder, which is then mixed.
- Measure the blood sugar before the injection and at 10 and 20 minutes.
- In some institutions, a physician must carry out the intravenous push.
- Glucagon causes the bowel to relax transiently, so the patient may complain of an altered sensation in the abdomen. Reassurance is all that is required.

Problem 6: zinc supplementation

Case

A 30-year-old female who you have treated for several years for AN complains of dry hands. On inspection, her hands are dry and have flakes of skin, but the rest of her skin appears normal. You ask her whether her taste has changed. She says no. On further questioning, she is using spices and salt on her food more than usual. Her serum zinc measurement is normal. You treat her with zinc gluconate 100 mg a day for two months; within two weeks the skin on her hands has returned to normal and within a month her taste has returned to normal.

Comment

The intake of zinc is largely dependent on milk products and seafood. Fiber binds zinc. The intake of zinc in AN is usually low, but deficiency usually takes months to years to occur. The serum zinc level is primarily dependent on the level of zinc-binding globulin and albumen in the blood and does not reflect the total body zinc storage. Additionally, testing for zinc deficiency by taste testing is unreliable.

The symptoms of zinc deficiency are dry, peeling skin on the palms and soles, change in taste (dysgeusia), impaired wound healing, and difficulty in healing skin infections. A possible zinc deficiency should be treated with oral zinc. A dose of 100 mg a day of zinc gluconate contains 14 mg of elemental zinc, which is the usual daily requirement of adolescents. Zinc supplementation can cause a copper deficiency if taken in doses about four times greater than this for many months. This is due to the competition of zinc and copper for the same route of absorption in the bowel.

Importantly, we have demonstrated that routine supplementation of zinc increases the rate of weight gain and recovery in AN. This is likely to be due to the modulation of neurohormones, especially in the amygdala.

Nursing implications

- About 2% of patients will complain of an upset stomach when taking zinc. This is best dealt with by giving the zinc with a meal.
- There are a few calories in each zinc gluconate tablet. Patients should be reassured that they are negligible. If the patient refuses to take zinc gluconate, another preparation of zinc may be available from the pharmacy, such as zinc sulfate. Whatever the formulation, ensure that the pharmacy substitutes the required 14 mg of elemental zinc.

PART III

Special issues

Chapter 8
Specific patient populations

8.1 Managing the chronic patient

Case

Cindy was a 40-year-old female with AN who I followed for 20 years, until her death. She had severe, unremitting, restrictive AN complicated by hyponatremia, hypokalemia, hypomagnesemia, an empyema of her lung, multiple bone fractures, renal failure, anemia, and, terminally, pneumonia and acute inferior myocardial infarction. Cindy had been admitted repeatedly over the years to various eating disorder units. She had tried and given up on many psychiatrists and psychologists, she was on chronic disability leave from her work, and within the last few years of her life she moved to an apartment in a suburb where she would eat very small amounts of food and have intermittent infusions of saline, potassium, and magnesium at home. Cindy had been emaciated for years, but she enjoyed helping others and always asked me about my children and would send them birthday presents. Although she could hardly hobble around with the use of a cane, she dressed in vividly colored glasses and maintained her dignity to the end.

Comment

Treatment of patients with chronic AN is widely misunderstood. As in many illnesses, the rate of recovery is variable. The average patient with AN may have the disorder for a few years, but many patients will continue to be anorexic for many years and some for life. Many physicians become confused when it appears that treatment does not work, then adopting a palliative care approach to the treatment of patients with "chronic" AN. This is tantamount to treating someone with asthma palliatively.

A full understanding of this perspective results in the following conclusions in chronic AN: (i) treatment of intercurrent medical and psychiatric conditions is still indicated; (ii) the treatment of malnutrition continues to be limited only by a continuing risk–benefit trade-off; (iii) focus on improved quality of life through rehabilitation; and (iv) as in asthma, AN may remit at any time in its course. Clinical remission in chronic AN usually occurs due to sociological change (e.g. divorce, death of a parent, decision to change careers) or because the patient simply becomes tired of being burdened with AN.

All patients with AN can recover – and some recover decades into their illness. However, while the patient continues to suffer from chronic AN, the important mode of treatment is a rehabilitation model.

Patients with chronic AN have ongoing signs and symptoms of protein-calorie malnutrition. They will have thinning of the hair, dry and yellow skin, decreased ability to focus the eyes, shortness of breath on exertion, decreased exercise capacity, repeated dysrhythmias, dizziness on standing, weakness, tiredness, hypothermia, muscle cramps, and decreased memory and concentration. In addition, they will suffer from progressive osteopenia, which will cause repeated fractures; these start off as stress factors and later become symptomatic fractures of the spine and lower extremities.

Chronic AN is associated with social isolation, an inability to work and learn, and diminished functional activity, including with family and friends and at work. Depending on the level of debilitation, the patient may be reclusive, living in a small apartment and isolated from their family, or they may be a thin individual with significant weight and shape concerns but who is fully integrated into their family, work, and society. Clearly, the rehabilitation goal is to move a patient with AN from the former to the latter situation.

The overall goals in following a patient with anorexia are:

- To prevent death by monitoring depression, actively preventing suicide, building rapport, searching for psychological comorbidity that might prevent improvement or diminish quality of life, helping to set goals for rehabilitation, and continuing to celebrate life with the patient at every visit.
- Medically, the frequency of follow-up varies, depending on the degree of illness, from every week to every three months. The weight, blood pressure, and heart rate should be taken. An inquiry regarding mood and plans should be taken, and goals should be established. If the patient is losing or gaining weight, then potassium, magnesium, and phosphate levels should be measured. If the weight is unchanged, this is not necessary. If there is significant deterioration in physical symptoms, then a systemic inquiry and physical examination with laboratory measures selected based on symptoms (often

to include hemoglobin, electrolytes, creatinine, AST, alkaline phosphatase, magnesium phosphate, vitamin B12, and ferritin) should be performed.

The physician should concentrate first on physical complaints. Chronic anorexics find it much easier to talk about physical concerns. Treatment of physical problems is easily accepted and appreciated, and this increases rapport. Treatment of urinary incontinence (which commonly occurs in chronic AN), careful care of feet and toes, and prevention of osteopenia with calcium and vitamin D supplements should all be considered. Use of the oral contraceptive pill to continue menstruation and potentially to increase bone mass should be discussed. In the authors' opinion, this is a two-edged sword, as medication treatment of osteopenia may be taken as a reason to focus less on nutrition.

Psychologically, focus on rehabilitation and quality of life. Any comorbid condition, such as a history of sexual abuse, substance abuse, or depression, should be sought and may require long-term treatment before other psychological gains are possible. If motivational enhancement therapy is available, then patients should be encouraged to undertake it. The primary physician should use a narrative approach in most cases. This focuses on discussing the patient's life not according to their daily miseries but in the context of how someone would want to retell their story. The narrative approach should focus in particular on how the patient's life could be improved to make the story more to the patient's liking. Often, it is useful to refocus the patient on their life by pretending it is a movie and changing the ending or episodes of the movie as they would if they were directing it.

One must be very careful regarding the involvement of the family in the treatment of chronic AN. Other family members often hold powerful feelings of guilt and anger towards the anorexic. The anorexic patient may also be ostracized from their family. Therefore, any discussions with family members are best done at the patient's request and with the patient present. As a primary physician, these are often in the form of family interventions. For example, the patient may wish to change their place of residence, apply for disability insurance, or discuss their position in the family. A physician can act as a mediator for the patient and explain the patient's disease in the context of a process for which chronic rehabilitation is necessary. It is of immense importance that the primary physician respects the right of privacy of the patient. This is particularly difficult in the setting of a family physician who has treated the entire family for years. It is our practice, and advice, that all patients who reach the age of majority be treated as independent adults – regardless of their health or place of residence. All parties – the patient, their family, and other hospital staff – must be aware of this policy, otherwise patient confidentiality will likely be breached and the patient's trust lost forever.

Medically, there are no medications other than food that are of absolute necessity in chronic AN. Some patients will accept ciproheptadine, which can be given at a dose of 4–16 mg at bedtime to increase fatty mass somewhat.

The use of chronic exercise in AN has been controversial. However, our work in the use of yoga in hospital and with a graded exercise program out of hospital to focus on breathing, stretching, and gradual incorporation of exercise to try to increase lean body mass and maintain bony mass is gaining acceptance. Paradoxically, exercise may decrease with a very gradual introduction of minimal activity in the patient with chronic AN. Certainly, if the physician simply proscribes activity, this is likely not to be accepted by the patient.

Indications for consultation in chronic anorexia nervosa

- Specific complaints, such as osteoporosis, chronic pain, and depression.
- Need for improved quality of life: weakness or other complaints that reduce quality of life must receive the usual investigation and treatment. This may require a rehabilitation approach.
- Motivation to change: during the course of the disease, many chronic patients will ask to engage in active therapy for their AN. This should be regarded as a great opportunity to involve them in therapy.

8.2 Diabetes mellitus

Case

A 19-year-old female with type 1 diabetes mellitus presents with confusion, depression, and greatly disordered eating.

Comment

The treatment of diabetes mellitus is often based on specialized diabetic education and follow-up, which are dependent on the results of the home blood glucose monitoring (HBGM) performed by the patient. The basic tenets of this treatment are to control activity, food intake, and insulin usage within certain boundaries, which can be varied by the patient based on the HBGM. It is easy to see why patients with AN will be controlled poorly and confound standard treatment plans and staff. This can impair rapport between the patient and the health care professionals, to the point where the patient is no longer followed adequately. More recently, as diabetologists have come to understand that about one-third of "brittle" diabetics are eating disordered diabetics, they have become allies of eating disorder clinics. This notwithstanding, sending an eating disordered patient to a diabetic clinic as initial care is not useful, so what is the preferred management?

- Outpatient treatment should be begun by a diabetologist in their office (not the diabetic clinic) and the eating disorder clinic.
- Focus on building rapport, correcting deficiency states, and setting goals.
- Admit the patient to an inpatient eating disorder unit for one to three weeks, initially with the goal of supporting eating and regulating activity and insulin usage.
- Activity during the inpatient unit should be planned by an occupational therapist to match normal activity out of hospital. Diet should match the planned discharge diet.
- The patient must perform blood sugar monitoring and insulin administration with the nurse supervising at all times.
- Cognitive function will usually improve markedly over the first two weeks as the fluctuations in blood sugar decrease and some degree of nutritional recovery is achieved.
- Discharge home with follow-up by the same diabetologist at least twice a week and pending plans for readmission, optimally to a day program.

Complications of diabetes mellitus that are hastened by an eating disorder

- *Small vessels:* retinopathy, renal failure, poor skin blood supply.
- *Large vessels:* stroke, heart attack, peripheral vascular disease, renal artery disease.
- *Metabolic:* hypoglycemia, with loss of consciousness; ketoacidosis, with reduced level of consciousness and risk of death.
- *Infection:* prone to bacterial infection; infections of feet and legs can progress rapidly, leading to amputation.

Management of diabetes mellitus in the patient with an eating disorder: some basics

- *Education:* all patients must attend a diabetic clinic for teaching.
- *Diet:* there must be an adaptation for eating disorders of the diabetic diet.
- *Exercise:* regular exercise must be maintained during regulation of the diabetes. Diabetic control depends on the effects of diet, exercise, and insulin together. Stress also changes diabetic control.

- *Insulin:* the insulin regimen should be managed by agreement between the patient and a diabetologist. We recommend that the diabetologist provides long-term follow-up.
- *Monitoring:* it is essential to monitor blood sugar four times a day during early treatment. Testing should be done by the patient, with supervision by a nurse.

Nursing instruction for patients with eating disorders and who have diabetes mellitus

- Supervise blood glucose monitoring and recording.
- Supervise insulin administration.
- The exercise routine of the diabetic will be designed to match their outpatient exercise. This is necessary for proper diabetic control. Educate other patients and staff as necessary.

8.3 Geriatrics

Case

A 72-year-old female with a long history of AN complicated by bowel complaints and osteoporosis is sent to you for advice about her severe back pain associated with multiple compression fractures of her vertebrae.

Comment

About half of those suffering from AN will not recover. Of these, some will live on to old age. Often, patients have adopted a lifestyle with which they are happy, until physical complications become incapacitating.

The most frequent long-term complication relates to bowel dysfunction, while the most incapacitating relates to bone fractures and pain. For specifics on the bowel and bones, see Sections 4.6, 4.9, and 5.10; what follows focuses on the special approach in the geriatric patient.

- Build trust and rapport in the context of an agreement about what the individual goals of the patient are. Usually, these goals are related only to the physical complaint at hand and do not relate to a change in eating or weight.
- Assess for coexistent psychological comorbidity, such as depression. The presentation of the patient at that particular time may relate as much to a change in affect as to a change in the physical complaint.

- Perform the history, physical examination, and laboratory tests with special attention to those disorders that are more likely to occur in the older patient. Deficiencies that take decades to occur, such as selenium and vitamin A, may have occurred by this age. Hypothyroidism, atherosclerosis, and cancer are also much more common in elderly patients.
- The dosages of medications must be adjusted downward, as in all geriatric patients.
- Geriatric patients have impaired recognition of sensations such as thirst and cold. Thus, they are more likely to become dehydrated during treatment.

Nursing implications for geriatric patients with anorexia nervosa

The goals of treatment for geriatric patients are similar to those for patients with other long-term diseases: rehabilitation and treatment of acute intercurrent disease.

- Depression may be harder to diagnose in the geriatric patient. Continue to observe for signs of depression.
- Have a higher index of suspicion of medication side effects because geriatric patients are more prone to them.
- Geriatric patients have impaired recognition of sensations such as thirst and cold. Monitor for adequate fluid intake and for hypothermia.

8.4 Males

Case

A 45-year-old male lawyer presents with incapacitating back pain. He has had AN for 20 years, but he has continued to practice and function well. He wants treatment to maintain his function.

Comment

AN is much more common in males than admissions to eating disorder units would indicate. Most males do not seek standard treatment for a variety of reasons, including the female orientation of treatment, the label of eating disorders as a female illness, the concern that they will be labeled as gay, and the medical acceptance in men of low body fat as normal or even laudable.

- Provide information indicating that eating disorders are common in men (especially male athletes), that there are treatment facilities that have great experience with males with eating disorders, and that eating disorders do not reflect sexual orientation. Having said this, there are some AN males who are gay and, especially among teens, who have uncertainty about their sexual orientation. Great sensitivity, acceptance, and knowledge of the issues involved are necessary to avoid irreparable damage to rapport.

- Offer the patient general eating disorder treatment. If he refuses treatment, offer him access to eating disorder specialists who have special expertise in treating males with eating disorders.
- Male anorexics are usually focused on the body shape of a weightlifter, being heavily muscled, especially in the upper body. Determine what your patient's ideal of body image is. It may require a high-protein, high-calorie diet to achieve.

Nursing implications

- Males have the same right to treatment as females.
- The treatment team often meets to discuss in advance the programmatic impact of a male patient. The team may unknowingly adopt a protective stance towards the female patients, who may have undergone sexual abuse or rape at the hands of a male. Care must be taken during these discussions to protect the confidentiality of the male patient both within the treatment team and from other patients.
- Male anorexics usually idealize the "V" shape of a weightlifter.

8.5 Overdose

Case

An 18-year-old female with a history of AN and major depression is brought into the emergency department by ambulance after her parents found her unconscious on the floor of her bedroom.

Comment

An overdose in AN should be treated as any other overdose. Certain issues however, should be stressed:

- There are a number of causes of unconsciousness in AN (see Section 5.5). Therefore, other causes of unconsciousness, especially hypoglycemia, hyponatremia, postictal state, and cardiac dysrhythmia, must be considered to coexist with the overdose.

- Patients with AN often receive and stockpile numerous medications obtained from many physicians over long periods of time. It cannot be presumed that the overdose is a single drug or that it is a recently prescribed drug.
- Coexistent vitamin and mineral deficiencies, drugs taken therapeutically, and malnutrition increase the risk of drug interactions and toxicity during treatment of overdose.
- Patients admitted for overdose are prone to suffering complications from the feeding syndrome because they have often been doing poorly nutritionally, may be non-compliant with vitamin and mineral supplements, and are managed in the intensive care setting without knowledge of the dangers of feeding.
- Patients with AN are prone to aspiration because they have muscle weakness, often have an incompetent lower esophageal sphincter, and have impaired intestinal peristalsis.

Nursing implications

- Monitor the blood glucose because unconsciousness after an overdose in AN can be caused by hypoglycemia.
- Record any information from friends or relatives about drugs or medications that the patient may have kept or had access to. AN patients often receive and stockpile numerous medications obtained from many physicians over long periods of time.
- Guard against aspiration. Aspiration is more likely to occur in overdoses in patients with AN because they often have an incompetent lower esophageal sphincter and have impaired intestinal peristalsis.

8.6 Pregnancy

Case

A 24-year-old female during recovery becomes pregnant whilst anorexic. Although not fully recovered, she is working, is living with her husband, and has required follow-up with decreasing frequency. She presents asking whether she and her baby are safe, whether she needs to be managed differently now that she is pregnant, and whether there will likely be problems after delivery.

Comment

Females with AN usually present with amenorrhea of variable duration. The amenorrhea can persist for six months or longer after weight recovery. Females often ovulate without menstruation, and they may therefore be fertile without being aware of this. Most pregnancies occur during recovery. During this phase, patients should be warned to use contraception if they do not want to become pregnant or if it is felt unadvisable medically. A pregnancy test should be performed as soon as pregnancy is considered. This should be done by the family physician, and consent should be obtained so that the eating disorder clinic can be notified immediately of the results. If the patient is pregnant (Figure 8.1):

- Assess the level of depression and suicidality.
- Reassess all medications, regarding their risk in pregnancy, and stop all those that should be stopped.
- A thorough history, physical examination, and laboratory tests must be performed.
- The patient should be assessed and followed by an obstetrician or family doctor as a high-risk pregnancy.
- Eating disorder follow-up should be weekly for a few weeks and then reduced to monthly if the patient is stable.
- A dietitian should assess the diet and nutrient supplements during pregnancy.

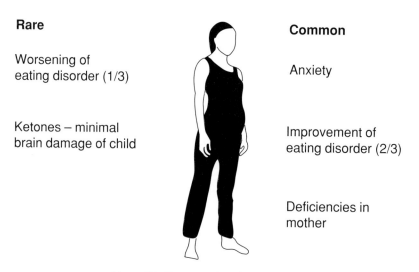

Rare

Worsening of
eating disorder (1/3)

Ketones – minimal
brain damage of child

Common

Anxiety

Improvement of
eating disorder (2/3)

Deficiencies in
mother

Figure 8.1. Pregnancy in eating disorders.

- A psychiatric or psychological reassessment should be performed with follow-up visits depending on need.
- Antepartum and postpartum mothers often have great concern about the effect that their eating disorder will have on their child. Children of anorexic mothers are often aware and take on a caregiver's role to the mother within the first few years of life. The children often develop disordered eating and body image. Therefore, psychological support for the mother, and later the child or family, is imperative.

Nursing implications for pregnancy in anorexia nervosa

- Most patients with AN who become pregnant do very well during pregnancy. The delivery is usually normal and the child is usually healthy.
- Prenatal care should be conducted routinely. If admission to hospital is required, it is best done on the prenatal ward, rather than the eating disorder ward, even if the issues are eating and weight gain. The chance of success is much greater under the normalizing influence of the prenatal ward. The eating disorder team can provide any additional specialized treatment on the prenatal ward.
- Antepartum and postpartum mothers often have great concern about the effect that their eating disorder will have on their child. Children of anorexic mothers are often aware and take on a caregiver's role to the mother within the first few years of life. The children often develop disordered eating and body image. Therefore, psychological support for the mother, and later the child or family, is imperative.

Chapter 9

Prepubertal children and younger adolescents

Based on the physical, psychological, and developmental characteristics of childhood and adolescence, significant differences and similarities may be expected from the adult population. This summary focuses on the negative biological effects and sequelae of eating disorders in children and adolescents. These may encompass effects on growth and pubertal development, and medical complications of different organ systems, including morbidity and mortality. All organs are affected by the protein-calorie malnutrition associated with AN. Similarly, the malnutrition seen with BN results in medical sequelae. Table 9.1 lists the medical complications commonly associated with eating disorders in children and adolescents. In addition, investigations and measurement strategies to assess the medical impact of eating disorders are discussed.

Adolescence may be defined using many different parameters. Chronological age is used most widely in the literature. For the purpose of this chapter, the terms "adolescent" and "youth" will refer to the age group between 11 and 19 years of age. From the philosophical point of view, adolescence may be defined as a time of change that encompasses not only biological changes but also major psychological and social adjustments.

A vast literature related to medical complications in patients with eating disorders already exists for the adult population, serving as an excellent source of reference for developing adolescents. Some of the previously highlighted differences between these two groups may be categorized based on the physiological hallmarks of adolescent development. Puberty may be defined as the sequence of anatomic and physiologic changes that result in physical maturity and the capacity to reproduce.

Prepubertal children and pubertal adolescents are faced with the possibility of stunted growth and delayed pubertal maturation, with irreversible and long-term effects on bone accretion, and structural and morphological changes of different organ systems, such as the brain. For the younger adolescent, acute

Table 9.1. *Eating disorders in children and adolescents: medical complications*

Complications	Anorexia nervosa	Bulimia nervosa
Fluids and electrolytes	Electrolytes are usually normal but may show low sodium, low chloride, low potassium and hypophosphatemia due to refeeding syndrome	Hypokalemic, hypochloremic, metabolic alkalosis with dehydration and vomiting Hyponatremia, diarrhea with laxative abuse Rarely mineral changes
Metabolic	Fasting hypoglycemia increases free fatty acids, with hyper/ hypocholesterolemia, hypercortisolism, osteopenia with decreased bone mineral density	Same as for AN Low zinc levels
Cardiovascular	Bradycardia, hypotension with orthostatic changes. EKG changes T wave, ST segment, and QTc abnormalities Sudden cardiac death, mitral valve prolapse, pericardial effusions, congestive cardiomyopathy, refeeding edema	Same as for AN Ipecac cardiomyopathy Pedal edema
Pulmonary	Decreased FEV_1, rib fractures, subcutaneous emphysema, pneumomediastinum	Bradypnea, aspiration pneumonitis
Gastrointestinal	Constipation, delayed gastric emptying, acute gastric dilatation, dyspepsia Transaminitis, decreased ALP Superior mesenteric artery syndrome, pancreatic dysfunction	Parotid swelling, palate lacerations, impaired taste, enamel erosion, increase caries, periodontal disease Gastroesophageal reflux, gastric and duodenal ulcers, esophageal tearing and perforation, acute gastric dilatation

(cont.)

Table 9.1. (cont.)

Complications	Anorexia nervosa	Bulimia nervosa
		Hyperamylasemia, pancreatitis
		Paralytic ileus, constipation, cathartic colon, rectal bleeding
		Gallbladder stones
Renal	Abnormal renal function test, with elevated urea and creatinine, changes in urinary concentration, decreased glomerular filtration rate, polyuria	Same as for AN Kaliopenic nephropathy, pyuria, hematuria
Endocrine	Amenorrhea Low LH, FSH, estradiol, TSH, T_3, and T_4 Increased reversed T_3 High cortisol and growth hormone levels, erratic antidiuretic hormone secretion, low peripheral catecholamines	Menstrual irregularities, polycystic ovaries
Hematological	Anemia, leukopenia, thrombocytopenia, bone marrow hypocellularity, low ESR	Anemia secondary to blood loss
Immunological	Decreased levels of complement factors	
Neurological	CT, MRI, PET scan abnormalities. Metabolic encephalopathy, with seizures	Metabolic seizures
Dermatological	Brittle hair and nails, hair loss, yellowish skin due to hypercarotenemia, dry skin, lanugo hair	Russell's sign, muscle weakness

ALP, alkaline phosphatase; CT, computed tomography; EKG, electrocardiogram; ESR, erythrocyte sedimentation rate; FEV, forced expiratory volume; FSH, follicle-stimulating hormone; LH, luteinizing hormone; MRI, magnetic resonance imaging; PET, positron-emission tomography; T3, triiodothyronine; T4, thyroxine; TSH, thyroid-stimulating hormone.

medical complications may pose a particular risk, based on a lack of adaptation to the major changes associated with abnormal eating behaviors seen in adults.

In contrast to anorexics, adolescents with BN or BED often appear physically healthy, with few symptoms and signs of illness. A subset of these patients is overweight and may present for advice on dieting. Furthermore, a large proportion of patients with AN also use vomiting and purging to increase weight loss. This combination is particularly dangerous. Such patients should be interviewed carefully about eating habits. Because binge eating is often done secretively, most patients will not provide this information unless asked specifically. In addition, the associated behaviors of purging and laxative, diet pill, diuretic, and ipecac abuse are often concealed from the health care worker. Such patients may present for medical care with non-specific complaints of feeling bloated, heartburn, constipation, or swelling of the hands and feet. The diagnosis can easily be overlooked if the physician misses these subtle clues.

9.1 Anthropometric assessment in children and adolescents

There is currently no single method that determines accurately an ideal body weight or a target weight for a child or adolescent who is struggling with an eating disorder. Most arguments in this regard state that conventional methodology that relates weight to age, sex, and height does not take into account ethnic differences and the inability to distinguish lean body mass from fat mass. In this section, a review of the current methods used to evaluate nutritional status of patients and to predict healthy weight ranges follows.

The most recent growth charts have been developed from the Third National Health and Nutrition Examination Survey carried out between 1988 and 1994.

During puberty, and due to different patterns of growth related to growth velocity, the best way to estimate growth patterns is by using standardized growth velocity tables. To this end, Tanner and Davies have developed normative standards, based on height and height velocity for North American children and adolescents from longitudinal data. A note of caution when interpreting a measurement that falls outside the third to fifth percentile when plotted against a standardized growth chart: these measurements are clearly not valid, and in this case it is recommended to consider using standard deviation scores (SDSs). Lastly, a note of caution when plotting an adolescent who is above the 75th percentile for height in standardized (weight for age and height for age) growth charts: a corresponding weight centile may exceed the appropriate weight for height by up to 20 kg when compared with height.

9.2 Body mass index

BMI is a method used to express the relationship between height and weight at any given age, for both genders. The Quetelet index is defined as the weight in kilograms divided by the square of the height in meters (BMI $= kg/m^2$). A basic failing of this method is the fact that even though it measures weight against height, it does not differentiate between fat or lean mass. Hammer and colleagues published standardized percentile curves of BMI for white children and adolescents, using data from the First National Health and Nutrition Examination Study in the USA from 1971 to 1974. Standards have been developed and published for both genders for ages 10–22 years by the American Medical Association. More recently BMI-for-age charts have become available from the National Center for Health Statistics from the Centers for Disease Control (CDC) in the USA.

9.3 Body composition

Assessment of body composition is of pivotal importance in the growing adolescent and is of great clinical value in the setting of patients suffering from eating disorders. Indirect estimation of the different body compartments may be undertaken by isotope dilution methods, electrophysiologic measurements, imaging, and anthropometric assessment.

Lean body mass (LBM) is defined as fat-free mass and comprises the active metabolic mass of the body; in this regard, total energy expenditure, intravascular blood volume, and maximum oxygen consumption are all functions of LBM. LBM may be estimated in several different ways. By measuring total body water or total body potassium, and based on the facts that LBM has a different density than fat and that neither electrolytes, nor water are bound by neutral fat, an estimation of LBM is possible.

In females, the LBM decreases from 80% of body weight at the beginning of puberty to about 75% at the end of puberty; this change is due mainly to the increase in total body fat from 15.7% to 26.7% once puberty is completed. For males, the changes are different, with LBM increasing from 80% to 90% by the end of pubertal development.

Subcutaneous accumulation of body fat takes place consistently during childhood and early adolescence. Limb accumulation of subcutaneous fat tends to decrease in both genders before the growth spurt. Males tend to lose fat tissue in their limbs during their peak height velocity or period of rapid growth. However, the accumulation of truncal subcutaneous fat remains relatively constant during this period and accounts for some of the weight gain that occurs in late puberty.

Pubertal changes are consistent and predictable, with an increase in total body fat for females and a decrease for males. For females, fat accumulation is a constant process, with an increase by the end of the growth spurt, and accounting for approximately 25% of female body weight. This accumulation of fat in females tends to predominate at the level of the lower trunk and thighs. For males, fat tissue accounts for approximately 12% of body weight by the end of puberty.

Skinfold measurement is by far the most widely and practicable method used to estimate subcutaneous fat. A note of caution relates to the fact that skinfold measurements need to be obtained by an experienced clinician who performs them regularly in order to decrease interobserver and intraobserver variability. The best instrument to obtain the measurements is the Harpenden caliper. By obtaining measurements at four different sites (biceps, triceps, subscapular, suprailiac), a well-trained examiner is able to use this method in a reliable fashion. Several different formulas have been developed for this purpose and have proven to be reliable when compared against more standardized methods, such as total body conductivity, bioelectrical impedance, total body potassium, total body dual-energy X-ray absorptiometry (DEXA), computed tomography (CT), and magnetic resonance imaging (MRI).

The upper-arm circumference is used to estimate muscle mass, providing relevant information in the growing adolescent suffering from malnutrition. The technique is simple and easily reproducible. A glass fiber tape that does not expand is applied perpendicular to the long axis of the arm. The patient relaxes and extends the arm down the side of their body, and a circumferential measurement of the arm, midway between the acromion and the olecranon, is taken. By taking this measurement and using normograms available, the mid-arm circumference may be estimated.

9.4 Medical manifestations in the adolescent

Bone

Bone accretion is one of the most salient features of puberty for both genders. Many factors are postulated to play a role in this process, including genetic, nutrition including somatic growth, weight, body composition, calcium and vitamin D intake, ethnic background, geographic location, exercise, and hormonal effects. A close interaction between the skeletal and endocrine systems is postulated. Growth hormone (GH), thyroid hormone and thyroxin, glucocorticoids, and sex steroids (estrogens, progesterone, testosterone, androstenedione, DHEA-S) modulate these changes by interfacing in the development of bone mass and by accelerating epiphyseal maturation and closure in bone.

Up to 50% in females and 67% in males of bone mass is attained during adolescence when followed longitudinally over a six-year period for magnitude and timing of peak bone mineral content velocity in relation to peak height velocity and menarche. A total of 53 young females, from two elementary schools in Saskatoon and Saskatchewan in Canada, and with a mean age of 10.06 years (range 7.97–13.26) were evaluated. The authors found that the timing of peak bone mineral content velocity and menarche were related closely and followed peak height velocity by approximately a year.

Martin and colleagues reported bone mineral and calcium accretion during puberty in both genders. They found that 32.2% of a total bone mineral content of 2200 g is calcium when measured in patients, and approximately 708 g of elemental calcium needed to be accumulated over a 20-year period to achieve this. The authors found that in males, the peak bone mineral content velocity was 320 g of calcium per year, corresponding to retention of 282 mg of calcium per day. For females, the peak bone mineral content velocity was 240 g of calcium per year, corresponding to retention of 212 mg of calcium a day. Based on published calcium absorption data, the authors estimated that males need a daily intake of calcium of 1335 mg and females require 1005 mg. Based on these findings, and the fact that North American adolescent diets are often deficient in calcium, the role of dietary calcium intake in children and adolescents with eating disorders remains of importance.

To date, the gold standard method for evaluating bone mass as it relates to tissue composition is DEXA. Two parameters in bone mineral density (BMD) measurement are important to consider: the T-score is the number of standard deviations (SDs) a subject's BMD is above or below sex-matched reference values in a given age range; the peak adult BMD follows a bell-shaped normal distribution curve. The Z-score is defined as the number of SDs that a subject's BMD is above or below age-, gender-, and ethnicity-matched mean reference values. The T-score is used for the assessment of fracture risk in postmenopausal women, and the Z-score is used to determine causes of low BMD. In evaluating child and adolescent BMD, the Z-score is used to determine how an individual's BMD compares with the expected BMD, based on published reference data. Other methods used to measure BMD include quantitative ultrasound and broadband ultrasound attenuation (BUA). This technique uses the calcaneous, due to its high content of trabecular bone. Mughal and colleagues published normative data for patients using this technique. This method does not use ionizing radiation, but its utility in this setting has not been established. Quantitative CT and magnetic resonance techniques are under investigation for the purpose of measuring BMD. These also do not involve ionizing radiation and have the advantage of providing information about bone architecture.

The earlier an eating disorder affects a patient, and the longer it affects them during adolescence, the greater the impact on bone health, risk for osteopenia, and reduction of peak bone mass. Osteopenia is defined as a deviation of between one and 2.5 SDs below the mean peak bone mass (T-score) for age and gender in BMD. It is estimated that up to half of patients with AN may develop osteopenia. Bacharch and colleagues evaluated 18 adolescent females (age range 12–20 years) with AN and 25 control subjects. The authors found that in this population, where the illness had been present for less than a year in up to half of the patients, low BMI correlated with bone mass and was an important predictor in the reduction of bone mass.

Osteoporosis is characterized by low bone mass, increased fragility of bone tissue, and increased risk for bone fractures. The World Health Organization (WHO) has defined osteoporosis as a BMD measurement (T-score) of greater than 2.5 SDs below the mean for Caucasian postmenopausal women. A negative correlation between low BMD, age of onset of AN, presence and duration of amenorrhea, and endogenous cortisol excess has been reported in adult and adolescent females.

Osteopenia and bone health improve with nutritional rehabilitation, weight restoration, and the return to a normal physiology of the endocrine-skeletal homeostasis. A prospective study reported 15 adolescent females aged 16.7 ± 2.4 years with AN, in whom the BMD had been measured one year earlier. A second group of nine adolescent females aged 17.8 ± 2.4 years and who had recovered from anorexia during adolescence was also reported. The authors found that despite improvement in BMD, eight patients had osteopenia of the spine and whole body, and increased bone mass correlated with weight gain before resumption of menses.

The use of hormonal replacement therapy to foster bone mineralization in adolescent females with AN remains a controversial topic. To date, there is no report in the literature of a prospective, randomized, controlled trial of hormonal replacement therapy in a population of young adolescents and its effects on bone. No consensus has been achieved among health care providers about the use of hormonal replacement therapy adjunct to standard treatment in adolescent patients with AN. Robinson and colleagues reported results of a survey conducted in 1998 by members of the Society for Adolescent Medicine. The authors found that despite the paucity of evidence in the literature with regard to the effectiveness of hormonal replacement therapy in improving bone health, more than 75% of the survey respondents reported using hormonal replacement therapy in older adolescents, but they used it less frequently in younger patients.

More recently, the National Institutes of Health (NIH) has funded the pilot for a multisite study observing the effects of bisphosphonate treatment during nutritional rehabilitation in AN. This medication promotes bone mineralization and is used to treat osteopenia in a number of other diseases.

In summary, prevention of osteopenia and optimizing bone growth and mineralization in adolescents with AN may be achieved by a two-track approach. First, bone growth and mineralization can be increased by weight restoration (promoting development of the muscle–bone unit). Second, facilitating resumption of normal menstrual physiology can increase BMD. In adolescents with AN and whose diet does not provide adequate calcium and vitamin D, supplementation of the recommended dietary allowance (RDA) to a total daily intake of 1200–1500 mg calcium and 400 IU vitamin D is considered optimal. Moderation in weight-bearing exercise should be encouraged and resistance exercising should be promoted.

Fluid and electrolytes

Child and adolescent patients with AN restrictive type frequently have normal serum electrolyte values. The cardinal feature associated with fluid and electrolyte disturbances in patients with eating disorders is intravascular volume contraction, which has been described well in adult, children, and adolescent populations. Dehydration in older children and adolescents is different from that in infants and young children. The common clinical picture seen in infants and younger children, including dry lips and mucous membranes, sunken eyes, crying without tears, and poor skin turgor, is rarely present in patients with AN. Vital sign instability with abnormalities in heart rate and blood pressure and skin manifestations are seen more commonly. Serum sodium tends to be in the upper limit of normal range, and blood urea nitrogen (BUN) and creatinine are usually elevated, despite a low muscle mass, representing a state of intravascular volume contraction.

Due to the adaptive mechanism to starvation, most malnourished patients present with bradycardia and hypotension, dry skin, cold hands and feet, and acrocyanosis (purplish discoloration of hands and feet). Patients with AN and chronic intravascular volume contraction rarely present with a heart rate above 60–80 beats per minute. In the case of normal or elevated heart rate associated with low systolic blood pressure (80–70 mm Hg), clinicians should be alert to these signs and act appropriately in terms of rehydration. It is accepted widely that aggressive rehydration in patients with AN and moderate to severe dehydration is not indicated, since it may precipitate cardiovascular collapse and heart failure.

Patients with BN commonly present with the well-described triad of hypokalemic, hypochloremic, and metabolic alkalosis associated with intravascular volume contraction and secondary compensatory hyperaldosteronism related to self-induced vomiting. Unpredictability of these metabolic changes makes serial measurement of serum samples to evaluate fluid and electrolyte status necessary, since predicting these abnormalities solely on the grounds of self-reported clinical information is not reliable. These patients often have orthostatic changes in blood pressure and heart rate, indicating intravascular volume depletion. Laxative use is the next most common compensatory behavior after self-induced vomiting in adolescents, with diuretic use and other purging methods being present less frequently. Patients who use laxatives often have decreased serum magnesium.

Serum phosphate levels fall in some patients during nutritional rehabilitation. This occurs in the first week of refeeding in about one-quarter of patients. Hypophosphatemia is the most dangerous manifestation of the refeeding syndrome, a well-known complication of nutritional rehabilitation in AN. Zinc deficiency that corrects during refeeding has been described. In addition to these electrolyte changes, deficiencies of other micronutrients have also been observed. Thiamine may be deficient.

Cardiovascular

Mortality rates associated with eating disorders are the highest among psychiatric disorders, with sudden death resulting from ventricular arrhythmias being responsible in up to 50% of the deaths. Cardiovascular changes were reported as "general depression of the circulatory function in previously normal young men with vigorous limitation of food intake" by Brozek and colleagues. In this article, the authors review the hemodynamic changes during starvation states and after refeeding and its effects on the cardiovascular system. They concluded that the increase in body weight and basal metabolic rate placed considerable strain on the cardiovascular system. Additional stress on the myocardium results from electrolyte abnormalities, hypothermia, and autonomic nervous system instability. These changes in association with hypophosphatemia are recognized as the refeeding syndrome and account for the mortality seen in early nutritional rehabilitation in AN.

Palla and Litt, in a retrospective chart review, reported cardiovascular changes as the most frequent abnormalities in a study of 65 subjects aged

10–20 years. These included bradycardia, hypotension, and abnormalities in electrocardiographic conduction, with prolongation of the corrected QT interval (QTc). More recently, a matched case–control study of electrocardiographic findings in adolescents (mean age 15 years) with eating disorders showed that a normal QTc interval on initial evaluation of an adolescent with AN does not correlate with disease severity, and that this finding should not falsely reassure clinicians. The authors suggest that relative bradycardia and decreased amplitude of the R-wave in V^6 are more useful electrocardiographic markers of disease severity in patients with AN, since these findings correlate significantly with lower BMI.

The mechanism of bradycardia in AN remains unclear, although it may be due to impaired autonomic function. Early reports are contradictory in relation to cardiovascular findings in adolescent and young adult patients with AN, with adaptive mechanisms to the starvation being postulated as the cause of cardiovascular changes.

Kollai determined cardiac vagal tone by measuring changes in the R-R interval on electrocardiograms in response to cholinergic blockage in a group of 11 adolescents (mean age 13. 6 ± 1.8 years) and in 11 age- and height-matched controls. The authors concluded that bradycardia in adolescents with AN was the result of vagal hyperactivity, and that enhanced baroreflex sensitivity likely contributed to the generation of excess vagal activity.

Kreipe and colleagues reported the use of power spectrum analysis (PSA) in evaluating autonomic dysfunction in adolescents with AN. Eight older adolescents (mean age 18.6 ± 3.9 years) and eight control subjects (mean age 20.9 ± 5.7 years) were studied; heart rate variability in the supine and standing positions at evaluation and after two weeks of nutritional rehabilitation was measured. The results indicated decreased sympathetic modulation of heart rate with postural changes. The authors suggest that PSA is a useful non-invasive method for monitoring autonomic control of heart rate in hospitalized patients with AN.

In addition, it is likely that cardiac function is also compromised from the effects of hypoglycemia and hypothermia that accompany protein-calorie malnutrition in AN.

Bingeing and purging behaviors have a significant impact on the cardiovascular system due to several mechanisms. The constant changes in intravascular volume, and the ongoing alterations in homeostatic balance related to electrolyte and metabolic derangements commonly seen in patients with BN, contribute to these changes. The putative effect of ipecac on the myocardium remains a concern in patients with eating disorders, despite efforts to regulate its availability. Emetine is the active alkaloid component in ipecac. Biochemical studies have demonstrated that emetine inhibits the oxidative activity of the citric acid cycle, and may also selectively damage myocardial mitochondria by impairing cellular respiration, carbohydrate metabolism, and protein synthesis. This results in myofibrillar degeneration and myocytolysis, leading to severe contractile dysfunction.

Endocrine

The endocrine changes observed in AN have been characterized well. Muller and Locatelli have reviewed the interface between malnutrition and pituitary function in AN in human and animal models.

Delayed puberty is one of the cardinal features of AN during adolescence. It is defined by a delay of more than two SDs beyond the mean for age and gender. The definition gender is as follows:

Females:

- Absence of breast development beyond 13.4 years of age.
- Absence of pubic hair development beyond 14.1 years of age.
- Absence of menarche by 16 years of age.
- More than five years elapsed between breast development and menarche.

Males:

- Absence of testicular growth (>2.5 ml) by 13.7 years of age.
- Absence of pubic hair development beyond 15.1 years of age.
- More than five years elapsed from initiation to completion of testicular growth.

An absence of progression through expected sexual maturity rating stages applies to both genders.

Important aspects of evaluating an adolescent with delayed puberty in the setting of an eating disorder include obtaining:

- *History*: growth records with previously recorded heights and weights; family history of linear growth, including parental and sibling height measurements; pubertal development from both parents, including information related to paternal puberty, and maternal and sisters' age of menarche. Other information related to standard medical history, with past medical, psychosocial, and systems review.
- *Complete physical examination*: measurement of vital signs and anthropometric parameters (height, weight, BMI, height/weight ratio; consider upper–lower body segmental ratios, arm span, body composition measurements by

skin folds). Evaluate sexual maturity rating. General physical examination, including genital examination to evaluate development of secondary sexual characteristics; neurological examination, including cranial nerves; examination of skin and hair; palpation of the thyroid gland; abdominal examination.

Primary amenorrhea is defined as the absence of menarche by 16 years of age in the presence of normal acquisition of pubertal developmental milestones. The investigation of this pathologic state should follow similar guidelines to those described for delayed puberty. (For a more detailed description of the assessment of an adolescent with primary amenorrhea, refer to Polaneczky, M. M. and Slap, G. B. Menstrual disorders in the adolescent: amenorrhea. *Pediatr. Rev.* 1992; **13**:43–8.) The progesterone challenge is a common method used to evaluate an adolescent with primary amenorrhea. Oral medroxyprogesterone acetate is administered in a dose of 5–10 mg daily for five to ten days. A withdrawal bleed should occur two to seven days later. This indicates the presence of endogenous estrogens, related to ovarian function, in the setting of a normal hypothalamic-pituitary-ovarian axis and a functional uterus.

The presence of amenorrhea in an adolescent female should prompt the clinician to evaluate other possible causes. Pregnancy, even though a rare event in young females with AN, needs to be excluded by obtaining a detailed clinical history, including health-risk behaviors and, more specifically, sexuality issues. Adolescents with BN seem to engage in more health-risk-taking behaviors than females with AN. A possible explanation for this phenomenon is the impulsive nature of the illness.

Amenorrhea is found in all postmenarchal females with AN according to DSM-IV criteria, and it is considered one of the clinical criteria for establishing diagnosis. This secondary amenorrhea is hypothalamic in origin and is due in part to suppression of the hypothalamic-pituitary-gonadal axis. Other factors include stress and the additive effects of malnutrition, weight loss, starvation, and strenuous exercise. Golden and Shenker explored the role of central dopaminergic and opioid activity in the genesis of menstrual disorders by administrating metoclopramide (a central D2 dopamine receptor blocker) to ten newly diagnosed women with AN and ten healthy age-matched controls. The authors found that metoclopramide did not induce significant changes in LH in either group. The multifactorial nature of secondary amenorrhea in postmenarchal females has been described well. Halmi and colleagues in 1977 reported that between 50 and 65% of individuals with AN may develop secondary amenorrhea before weight loss and that amenorrhea may persist, despite attainment of a healthy weight range. Bryant-Waugh and colleagues reported in a 7.2-years (mean) follow-up study of children and adolescents with early-onset AN that

55% of recovered patients were having regular menstrual periods, 31% were amenorrheic, and 14% were having irregular periods. Lai and colleagues have reported similar findings in a group of children and adolescents: 50% of patients had primary amenorrhea and the other half had secondary amenorrhea, having reached a mean ideal body weight of 96.5% (range 90–108%). Half of the patients in each group resumed or started menstruating. The group with continued amenorrhea had a lower ideal body weight (mean 87.5%, range 76–96%). The authors concluded that standard body weight goals set for patients with AN may be too low, and that pelvic ultrasound may aid treatment.

Golden and colleagues reported results related to factors associated with resumption of menses a group of 100 adolescent females with a mean age of 16.9 years (range 12–24 years) followed for a two-year period. Resumption of menses was defined as two or more consecutive spontaneous menstrual cycles, and the treatment plan included medical, nutritional, and psychiatric interventions. Menses resumed at 9.4 ± 8.2 months after initial assessment and required an increase of 2.05 kg over the menstrual threshold (weight at which menses stopped). The percentage of standard body weight was 91.6 ± 9.1%, with 86% of patients resuming menses within six months of reaching this weight. At follow-up, a serum estradiol level of more than 110 pmol/l was associated with resumption of menses. The authors concluded that a weight of approximately 90% of standard body weight was the average weight at which resumption of menses occurred; this is a reasonable treatment goal weight, and serum estradiol levels at follow-up best assess resumption of menses.

The studies above show that in adolescents with AN, resumption of menses occurs at different body weights. The authors suggest the use of ancillary methods such as pelvic ultrasound; serum estradiol may be used to predict this significant landmark in the treatment of patients with eating disorders.

It is common to observe irregularities in the menstrual cycle in BN, with 30% of patients experiencing secondary amenorrhea. BN is associated with polycystic ovaries. The reason for this association is unknown, but it is hypothesized that insulin resistance may develop due to the eating behaviors associated with the illness, namely bingeing and purging. Jahanfar and colleagues evaluated 94 adult twin females, and found that 42 subjects had polycystic ovaries by transabdominal ultrasound. The majority of women with polycystic ovaries have been reported to have abnormally elevated scores on tests of eating attitudes.

Hematological

Bone marrow hypoplasia and its implications in this population have been described. In children and adolescents with AN, the most commonly seen hematological changes are normal or marginally low hemoglobin, and hematocrit with abnormal erythrocyte indices, showing increased mean corpuscular volume (MCV), mean corpuscular hemoglobin (MCH), and mean corpuscular hemoglobin concentration (MCHC). These macrocytic changes are rarely associated with folate or vitamin B12 deficiency in this patient population, but they need to be considered. Other abnormalities include leukopenia and thrombocytopenia. All of these changes are reversible with weight restoration and nutritional rehabilitation.

Microcytic, hypochromic anemia due to iron deficiency is considered to be one of the most common nutritional deficiencies for growing adolescents, with a peak prevalence (3.5–14.2%) between the ages of 11 and 19 years for both genders. Iron-deficiency anemia is rarely seen in the initial stages of AN in female patients, possibly due to the protective effects of amenorrhea. When present, other causes of chronic blood loss, such as inflammatory bowel disease, malabsorptive syndromes and exudative enteropathy, parasitic infections, and underlying organic disorders of a chronic nature, need to be excluded. For adolescent males, the risk of iron-deficiency anemia may increase due to expanding blood volumes and muscle mass related to the growth spurt.

Anyan characterized the changes seen in erythrocyte sedimentation rate (ESR) and fibrinogen in patients with AN. Palla and Litt reported that a low ESR was common in their malnourished patients with anorexia. This parameter may be used to aid in the differential diagnosis of AN from other ominous causes of malnutrition (infectious processes, chronic inflammatory and systemic illnesses).

Microcytic, hypochromic anemia related to iron deficiency may be seen in females with BN due to secondary blood loss through the gastrointestinal tract and related to mucosal irritation and damage.

Neurological

A significant body of literature has discussed the connection between eating disorders, the nervous system, and the etiology of this illness. A variety of neurological abnormalities occur in adolescent patients with eating disorders, but to date there is no conclusive evidence that a central nervous system or, more specifically, a primary hypothalamic disorder is linked to the genesis of the illness.

A study group in AN sponsored by the WHO and Association Internationale pour la Recherche et l'Enseignement en Neurosciences met in 1993. The group looked at neuroendocrine and neurotransmitter abnormalities and neurological aspects, and proposed guidelines for future epidemiological research in the area of AN. The group stated:

- In humans, there are limited methods of assessing the serotoninergic system, but there is evidence that 5-hydroxytryptamine (5-HT) function is abnormal in patients with AN during and after recovery from the illness. By having a better understanding of the role of 5-HT function in AN, there may be better treatment options for this resistant disorder.
- Even though the neuroendocrine abnormalities of AN have been well described, there is no clarity regarding its role in the etiology or pathophysiology of the disorder. Biofeedback mechanisms and circadian hormonal rhythm disturbances are examples of the interface between the central nervous and the endocrine systems.
- The atrophy and enlargement of the cerebral ventricles described by neuroimaging techniques such as CT and magnetic resonance remain of unclear etiology. Malnutrition and dehydration alone do not explain the changes seen with these techniques. Positron-emission tomography (PET) holds the possibility of linking anatomical and functional abnormalities in the study of the role of the central nervous system changes in AN.

Early radiological investigations of the central nervous system in AN included cranial CT. Before the use of this modality of radiological investigation, Heinz and colleagues reported structural brain changes in patients with AN by pneumoencephalographic studies in 1961.

Enzmann and Lane reported abnormal enlargement of cortical sulci and subarachnoid spaces, as compared with a control group, in three adolescent females of 16, 14, and 15 years of age, and in one adult of 30 years of age. These females had lost 16–40 kg over six months to five years before CT. Heinz and colleagues, in the same periodical issue, presented a case report of two patients, a 15-year-old female with malnutrition due to AN and a nine-year-old boy with Cushing's syndrome. The two patients showed the CT abnormalities described previously, and in both cases these reverted after treatment. The authors postulated that the changes observed in the abnormal scans were possibly due to protein loss, fluid retention, or both.

In 1980, Nussbaum and colleagues reported 14 patients with AN, mean age between 14.1 and 15.7 (range 10–19) years old, with a weight loss of between 10 and 20% of their total body weight. The authors observed that there were two groups of findings: the abnormal group, which comprised three males and four females who had lost significantly more weight and in a shorter period of time, and the normal group, which was comprised of seven females. The authors also observed persistent cortical atrophy in two patients despite weight restoration.

Katzman and colleagues, in 1996, showed, using MR studies in adolescent females (age 15.2 ± 1.2 years) with AN, large total cerebrospinal fluid volumes and a cerebral gray and white matter total volume deficit. A correlation between cortisol levels and brain changes was also described in this group, with a relatively short duration of the illness. The same group of researchers showed a persistent gray matter volume deficit, but no deficit in white matter, in weight-recovered subjects with AN. These findings support the theories that AN has reversible and irreversible effects on the brain. The authors concluded that AN might have long-lasting and global effects on the brain.

Regional cerebral blood flow (rCBF) has been used to evaluate the possibility of a functional correlation with the structural brain alterations in patients with eating disorders. Krieg in 1989 studied a group of 12 female inpatients (age 21.3 ± 3 years old, range 16–27) with AN, evaluated their brain morphology by CT, and correlated it to rCBF at admission and after weight gain. The authors concluded "that regional cerebral blood flow studies by xenon-133 dynamic single-photon emission tomography (dSPECT) yield no suggestion that there was any reduced function of certain brain areas in AN."

Gordon used rCBF with single photon emission computerized tomography (SPECT) in children. The authors evaluated 15 children (age 8–16 years) who were less than 80% of body weight as expressed by assessing weight for height ratio. Thirteen patients had abnormal scans with hypoperfusion in the temporal lobe area, eight in the left and five in the right side; three follow-up scans in weight-recovered patients showed persistent abnormalities. The authors defined as abnormal a left-to-right difference of over 10% in the perfusion profile. This unilateral abnormality may be linked to an underlying biological substrate in the etiology of AN. Another 14 patients have been scanned since the original report, with 80% showing unilateral abnormalities.

Renal

Impairment of renal function occurs in AN from pre-renal and renal factors. In the former, dehydration and low circulating blood pressure and volume contribute to the pre-renal effects. Persistent and severe protein-calorie malnutrition results in a diffuse glomerular sclerosis. This is a non-reversible insult to the kidney, leading to a progressive decline in glomerular filtration rate and eventually renal failure if nutritional rehabilitation does not occur.

In persistent hypokalemia as a result of chronic vomiting or diuretic abuse, as in BN and AN patients who purge, vacuolation of the renal tubules has been observed, resulting in impaired tubular function, which affects fluid and electrolyte balance.

Hepatic

Non-alcoholic steatohepatitis (NASH syndrome) occurs in some patients with AN. Typically, the transaminase levels are in the several hundreds but not thousands. The raised enzyme levels persist for several weeks at the beginning of nutritional rehabilitation. These changes are usually asymptomatic and uncomplicated. Liver biopsies reveal a combination of micro- and macrovesicular steatosis. These changes resolve with nutritional rehabilitation.

Morbidity and mortality

AN in adults has the highest morbidity and mortality rate among psychiatric illness. Herzog and colleagues reported a 5.1% crude mortality rate in a naturalistic study in its eleventh year. Sullivan reported findings on a meta-analysis suggesting a 5.6% mortality rate per decade in AN. Some studies estimate that death rates of young women with AN are up to 12 times those of age-matched women in the community, and up to twice those of women with other psychiatric disorders. Hawley reported in 1985 results on 21 children and adolescents aged 13 years or younger at onset of the illness, with a mean follow up of eight years. A total of 19% of patients were male, with symptoms being present from 0.1 to two years (mean 0.7 years); no deaths were reported at follow-up. Other outcome studies have found an overall mortality rate of 3.2% (range 0–18%) for a total of 186 patients. Hsu reviewed 16 outcome studies published between 1954 and 1978 and found a similar range (0–19%) for the mortality rate.

Bryant-Waugh and colleagues conducted a long-term follow-up study (mean 7.2 years) in England of 30 children and adolescents with early-onset AN. Of the reported sample, 23 patients were females and seven were males, with a mean age of onset of the disorder at 11.7 years (range 7.7–13.2), and 20.8 years (range 14–30) at follow-up. The authors reported a good outcome in 60% of the sample. Ten patients remained moderately to severely impaired, and two died. Amenorrhea and menstrual abnormalities were prevalent in nearly 50% of the sample, and 25% of the patients required further admissions to hospital with associated psychiatric diagnoses.

Kreipe and colleagues reported results in 49 adolescents diagnosed with AN and admitted to an adolescent medical inpatient unit; the patients were followed for a mean period of 80 months. The Global Clinical Score scale was reported as the tool used to measure outcome variables. A total of 86% of patients had a satisfactory outcome, with a mean body weight at 96.1% of estimated standard body weight and resumption of menses in 80% of the patients. A total of 15 pregnancies occurred, with ten healthy newborns, two elective abortions, and three ongoing pregnancies at the time of the report. Of the sample, 25% had persistent daily food restrictions and 29% were struggling with binge eating behaviors. Self-induced vomiting was reported in 25% of the subjects.

Strober and colleagues reported no deaths, with a 76% recovery rate of a total cohort of 95 patients admitted to the specialty treatment program for AN at UCLA Neuropsychiatric Institute. In this study, the authors reported on the long-term course of AN in adolescents, with an age range at entrance to the study of 12–17 years and 11 months, and with illness duration ranging from eight to 88 months. Most (92.6%) patients were white, and most (89.5%) were female. The findings included a protracted time of recovery, ranging from 57 to 79 months depending on the definition of recovery. The authors point out that some of the limitations of the study include its selective nature, due to the specialty treatment aspects of the university medical center, and the follow-up interview methods.

9.5 Conclusions

Children and adolescents struggling with eating disorders face a number of medical complications that are different from those experienced in adulthood, due to developmental characteristics of younger patients. A better understanding of the nuances of the physiological processes involved in linear growth and pubertal development during the adolescent years may alleviate some of the irreversible long-term effects of patients struggling with eating disorders. To date, the effects of malnutrition on the developing body have been well documented and are clearly associated with the increase in morbidity seen in this patient population.

Prepubertal children and pubertal adolescents are faced with the possibility of stunted growth and delayed pubertal maturation, with irreversible and long-term effects on bone accretion, and structural and morphological changes of different organ systems, such as the brain. For the younger adolescent, acute medical complications may place these patients at risk of medical complications, based on lack of adaptation to the major changes associated with abnormal eating behaviors seen in adults with chronic eating disorders. Setting treatment goals for patients requires a comprehensive assessment and understanding of the particular individual's needs, based on their stage of development. To date, weight restoration and nutritional rehabilitation remain the cornerstones of the biological treatment for children and adolescents struggling with eating disorders, with a two-track approach and appropriate psychosocial interventions to achieve recovery from this devastating illness.

PART IV

The psychiatric and psychological perspective

Introduction

The purpose of this part of the book is different from that of the first half. Here, the aim is to provide information about the psychiatry, psychology, and sociology of AN and related eating disorders. It will discuss assessment, prevention, and psychological treatment, but it is not meant to be a definitive guide on these matters, as the first part is on medical treatment. The intended audience remains the same: health care workers of all disciplines who are involved in the care of patients suffering from AN or one of its related eating disorders. Others in the community may also find items of interest in the book – such as members of the legal profession, school teachers, welfare workers, and even parents, relatives, and friends of patients who have or have had these illnesses. However, because health care workers are the primary audience, the book contains much that is technical in medicine. No attempt has been made to explain or clarify the technicalities.

This part is concerned with the psychiatry, psychology, and sociology of eating disorders. For those health workers who have not been trained in mental health per se, it offers a review of the mainstream ideas of those psychiatrists and psychologists who have a particular interest in these illnesses. Because some of the concepts used in psychiatry and psychology are unfamiliar to other health care professionals, it includes some clarification of psychiatric and psychological terms. Mental health workers who work outside the area of eating disorders will probably not need these clarifications, but they may be interested in the way terms common to psychiatry and psychology in general are applied to this particular area of clinical work.

Chapter 10

Physical disease and mental illness: pathology and psychopathology

The implied dualism between body and mind may upset the good physician, who rightly sees the whole human being as their province of interest. "Disease" and "illness" are synonyms in the *Shorter Oxford English Dictionary*, one deriving from old French, the other from Gothic. Nevertheless, there is heuristic value in distinguishing between the two. It has been suggested that the word "disease" be reserved for a condition in which an abnormality of function has been brought about by a change in anatomy, histology, biochemistry, physiology, or molecular biology – in other words, an underlying pathology. Disease is a useful concept in all the biological sciences. Any organism may suffer from disease. Illness, on the other hand, is a social rather than a biological concept. It is appropriately applied only to human beings – one does not attribute illness to an earthworm, although one may be tempted to do so to a favorite dog. Illness indicates that the person affected is not as they should be – not behaving, or not thinking, or not feeling as they or other members of their community think is appropriate. Illness is merely one way of explaining this dissonance – others might include a cold wind blowing or because there has been a recent serious loss or trauma. Illness has specific social implications in that it conveys certain privileges and responsibilities to the ill person, e.g. they may be excused from attending work or school. On the other hand, the patient is expected to seek treatment and comply with it as long as it is reasonable.

Illness is often based on underlying disease, i.e. on there being a disease with a pathology of some type present, even if it is mild. In the case of physical illness, there is always presumption of an underlying disease, even if the latter has not been discerned. Those physical illnesses in which no consistent pathology has been identified despite intensive investigation – perhaps repetitive strain injury or chronic fatigue syndrome – are controversial. In psychiatry, most mental illnesses do not have discernible underlying pathology, although some do. (Dementia may result from many causes, including nutritional deficiencies. It may also be the result of a specific brain condition, such as Alzheimer's disease.) In other instances, a brain dysfunction is suspected but has not yet been proven, e.g. AN and major depression. In yet others, it would appear unlikely that the cause of the illness is other than a combination of experiential and constitutional factors, e.g. bereavement, post-traumatic stress disorder, BN. Eating disorders may fall between these two groups: there is reason to believe that severe AN may have an organic basis because of its strong familial aggregation and because several genes have been identified with respect to it. On the other hand, patients whose symptoms are explainable entirely by a contribution of overweight and reaction to social pressures to be thin may develop BN, BED, or the milder forms of EDNOS, but they are unlikely to have a brain disease.

Because of the lack of a definite pathology in respect to most mental illnesses, it has been necessary to develop another analogous construct to that of psychopathology. But psychopathology is merely an analogy to pathology. It is really very different from it, and these differences must be recognized explicitly. The psychopathology is not diagnostic for any mental illness. Thus, a patient with the diagnosis of schizophrenia may have depression, paranoid ideation, hallucinations, and loss of volition in their psychopathology. Similarly, a patient with AN may have overvalued ideas, obsessional thinking, anxiety, or depression in their psychopathology. The psychiatric diagnosis arises from the consistency of association of the various psychopathological features.

Chapter 11

Psychopathology and the mental status examination

A major difference between psychiatry and the other disciplines of clinical medicine is the complete dependence of the former on the mental state examination. Although the physical examination of the patient is always important in medicine, the mental status examination is absolutely fundamental to the concepts of psychiatry and to its clinical practice.

Psychiatry is concerned with mental illnesses. Some of these are based on underlying organic pathology, usually of the brain. The dementia that arises from thiamine (vitamin B1) deficiency is an example. In others, an underlying pathology is suspected but not yet proven, e.g. schizophrenia. For yet other psychiatric illnesses, it is generally accepted that no pathology exits and that the illness has arisen entirely from constitutional or experiential factors. Post-traumatic stress disorder and BN are examples. Because of the heterogeneity of psychiatric illnesses, the wide variation in their causation, and the inconsistency of their association with physical pathology, it is necessary to add another criterion to the description of any mental illness, i.e. the construct of psychopathology. Without the presence of a psychopathology, the distinction between mental illnesses and other presentations of statistical abnormality are entirely arbitrary. Thus, a person who uses laxatives on the instruction of their physician for a disorder of the bowels is quite different from a person who uses laxatives based on imaginary fears of becoming obese. It is not the use of laxatives that defines an illness; it is the mental processes that have led to its occurrence. These mental processes are identified by the mental state examination, which reveals the psychopathology.

Unlike the organs of the body, such as the brain, liver, and kidneys, the mind is an insubstantial concept, in that its functions cannot be measured by any physical means. They can be described only by reference to mental functions per se, i.e. by reference to a combination of the behaviors involved, the internal mental experiences that the patient describes, and whatever impairments

211

may be charted by careful questioning. Thus, psychopathology is entirely dependent on the mental state examination, not something independent of it, as pathology is independent of the physical examination. The so-called instruments used in psychiatry and psychology are not instruments in the same sense as the sphygmomanometer is an instrument to measure blood pressure or blood glucose levels are used to measure biochemical function. Psychological and psychiatric instruments are merely aspects of a mental state examination designed specifically to collect information in as objective and reliable a way as possible.

The reliance of psychiatry on the concepts of psychopathology are not acknowledged fully by all psychiatrists, let alone by their colleagues in other branches of medicine, the law, or the public in general. Just because Wernicke's encephalopathy is caused by a deficiency of thiamine does not mean that all the psychiatric symptoms of an eating disorder patient with thiamine deficiency are due to Wernicke's encephalopathy. The patient may also be depressed and require antidepressant medication. In respect to abnormalities of eating behavior, a diagnosis of food allergy can only be confirmed by blinded testing with food and placebo or controlled dietary manipulation. If this is not done, then one may infer either that some unknown allergy exists, which cannot be confirmed, or that the patient is feigning symptoms, especially if the real cause is a psychiatric illness such as AN that leads the patient to delude themselves into a genuine belief that they have an allergy.

Terms used in relation to psychopathology must not be given more authority than they warrant.

Anorexia nervosa is derived from the Latin meaning "without appetite." Yet patients with AN usually have a voracious appetite. Bulimia nervosa is derived from the Greek meaning "hungry as an ox." However, BN is not necessarily associated with great hunger; it is a habituation to a pattern of eating and purging.

There are several other issues that need to be explored to assist non-psychiatrists in understanding what psychiatrists mean. Psychopathology may refer to the form or the content of mental experiences. Formal psychopathology concerns itself with the way in which a symptom is experienced. Thus, there is a major distinction between the firmly held false belief that is termed a delusion, and is usually associated with a psychosis like schizophrenia but may be seen in AN, and the persistent, nagging doubt that a patient may hold despite their realization that it is probably unfounded, which is called an obsession, and which is also seen in anorexic patients. Content psychopathology refers to the dominant theme in the patient's mind, such as the gloomy thought, despondency, and despair of a severe depression, and the fear of weight gain that leads to the anxiety and abnormal behavior of AN. Form and content psychopathology are not consistently related to each other. For instance, an anorexic patient may move from having an overvalued idea as to the central importance of their weight to their life in general, through a stage of obsessive preoccupation with this idea that they have come to doubt, and finally to a delusional stance in which they accept the proposition unconditionally, to the extent that they are not able to alter their behavior despite overwhelming evidence that it is dominating their very existence and not leading to the happiness they seek but rather compounding their problems even further.

Another distinction in psychopathology is between the objective and the subjective. Objective psychopathology seeks to describe mental experiences in operational terms. Thus, a delusion is defined as a false belief, usually referring to the person themselves either as the subject or the object (i.e. being endowed with special qualities or deficiencies, or being the object of improbable influences, such as persecution by supernatural forces). Delusions are impervious to change by logical argument or by the demonstration of their false basis, and are usually persistent, although sometimes their exact content may be ephemeral. The distinction between a delusion and another unsubstantiated belief is often arbitrary and depends on the social and cultural context of the patient. Thus, a person raised in a strictly vegetarian home and who has strong beliefs about the importance of avoiding animal products may be thought to have an overvalued idea about food. But one who goes on to stubbornly refuse adequate sustenance to maintain their life, believing that they can survive without any significant energy intake and refusing any compromise, is more properly considered delusional. It is the impervious and intractable nature of the belief, and the manner in which it is held, rather than the content, that warrants the term "delusion."

Obviously, the distinction between psychiatric psychopathology and other human experiences that are unusual or generally rejected is both difficult and apparently arbitrary from the viewpoint of those who do not understand psychiatry or accept its basic principles. However, those who seek to dismiss psychiatric illness as imaginary must realize that to do so would be to reject the distinction between a deranged psychiatric patient who is not responsible for their actions and a person who is sane but acting in an abnormal way, perhaps under the influence of psychoactive drugs or a commitment to a cause such as terrorism. One cannot abandon the reality of one mental illness without rejecting all. So, there is a persistent dualism. In relation to a physical complaint such as abdominal cramping previously diagnosed as irritable bowel syndrome, the clinician must decide whether this is based on a physical pathology that has yet to be identified, whether it is really a mental illness, or whether it is simply imaginary or malingering. In respect to mental illness, recourse is made to a careful examination of the proposed psychopathology. Not only the objective psychopathology, but also the subjective psychopathology or phenomenology, must be examined, i.e. the actuality that the patient experiences. Thus, the usual definition of a delusion is that it is a fixed, false belief, impervious to logical argument and out of keeping with the patient's social and cultural context. A person cannot hold with conviction a belief that they realize is false. From the subject's point of view, a delusion is an idea that is held with such conviction that its truth seems impossible to deny. If it were false, then the whole world would be false. It is not a matter of being impervious to reason, but being something that cannot be subjected to reason. It is like the beliefs of a patient with AN about shape and weight rather than the misinformation under which a patient may present to lose weight for good cause.

Because of differences of this nature, it is difficult to reconcile psychiatric concepts of illness with medical concepts of disease. Another, equally important, distinction relates to causation. In relation to physical disease, we are concerned only with the explanatory cause: dementia in the anorexic patient is due to the disturbance of neural function caused by the nutritional deficiency. In psychiatric illness, we are concerned not only with the explanatory cause but also with understanding it. Thus, a patient with an eating disorder may have a pseudo-dementia due to severe accompanying depression rather than a true dementia per se.

Chapter 12

Psychopathology and phenomenology

The objective psychopathology of AN is difficult to label. It relates to an unwillingness to eat, a determination to be unnaturally thin, and evident contentment with being capable of refusing to eat and being emaciated. This has been termed a hysterical symptom, a phobia of weight gain, an obsession, a delusion, and an overvalued idea. Probably all of these terms are justified in patients at different stages of their illness. Patients are overwhelmed by concerns about their body and protest that they feel themselves to be fat even when they are actually emaciated. They are preoccupied with ways to reduce their weight further or, at the least, to prevent any weight gain. They appear genuinely terrified at the prospect of being overweight, and some patients state openly that they would rather be dead than fat. Although so extreme as to be pathological, such beliefs represent an exaggeration of the widespread concern about weight and shape that has become engendered in our society. In most patients with AN, these beliefs would best be termed "overvalued ideas." When they are held stubbornly despite overwhelming evidence that the behavior has become life-threatening, they are interpreted as delusions, in that the patient is no longer able to examine them rationally.

On to this core concern are imposed other psychological symptoms, many of which are known to be common in semi-starvation irrespective of cause (Table 12.1). These include depressed mood, irritability, social withdrawal, loss of sexual libido, preoccupation with food, obsessional ruminations and rituals, and eventually reduced alertness and concentration. Dysphoria is particularly important, being an integral feature of the illness. Many clinicians who make an inappropriate second diagnosis of a mood disorder do not appreciate this intimate association. In the past, the misdiagnosis of a mood disorder often led to the prescription of tricyclic antidepressant drugs, which pose physical dangers to the anorexic patient whose cardiac function might already be compromised. Nowadays, selective serotonin reuptake inhibitors (SSRIs) are more likely to

Table 12.1. *Common psychological symptoms of anorexia nervosa*

Caused or worsened by semi-starvation
  Depression
  Loss of concentration
  Preoccupation with thoughts of food
  Anxiety
  Labile mood (i.e. fluctuating from one extreme to another)
  Irritability
  Feelings of inadequacy
  Hypersensitivity to noise
  Obsessional thinking
  Increased perfectionism
  Social withdrawal so as to avoid situations that involve eating
  Depression and suicidal ideation
  Poor sleep quality (interrupted, fragmented, not restful)
  Compulsive behaviors

Likely pre-existing or unrelated to semi-starvation
  Low self-esteem
  Obsessional traits
  Tendency towards perfectionism
  Symptoms of depression, including low mood, feelings of guilt, feelings of
    helplessness, and hopelessness
  Obsessional and compulsive traits
  Symptoms of anxiety, including panic attacks

be used; these are certainly less dangerous, but there have been no objective studies of their value in treating the depression in these patients. Similarly, severe obsessional symptoms, usually relating to eating and food but sometimes of a more general nature, are common in AN patients. Often, but not invariably, these symptoms improve with weight gain.

The illness is associated with premorbid perfectionism, introversion, poor peer relations, and low self-esteem. The patient may be described as having been an attentive and helpful child, and whose current obstinate refusal to eat is all the more extraordinary because of their previous compliance. In the early stages, as the patient becomes increasingly preoccupied with dieting, they withdraw from peer relationships, concentrating on study or work to the exclusion of all other interests. Some patients, however, will have been extroverted and interactive, with outgoing personality profiles and a history of behavioral disturbance.

Patients react to efforts to alter their behavior with anger, deception, and manipulation, often inconsistent with their previous behavioral standards. With chronicity, they become absorbed by their illness, dependent on family or therapists, and restricted in their interests. The serious long-term effects of regression, invalidism, and social isolation come to dominate the clinical picture.

Many patients' emotional problems arise from separation anxiety and difficulties with identity. There is sometimes a "pathogenic secret," such as sexual abuse, which results in intense feelings of shame. Starving is a means of assuaging the pain and gaining control over the course of sexual development. The patient holds on to their emaciation as a form of self-realization and identifies with their wasted body.

Intense feelings of guilt are frequently, and paradoxically, present. Patients complain that they feel guilty if they eat or do not exercise, but they also feel guilty if they do. They relate these feelings to their extremely low self-esteem.

Although this pattern of disturbance imparts conformity to the psychiatric presentation, the underlying phenomenology and psychodynamic psychopathology are varied. Each patient needs to be understood as an individual. Comorbid substance abuse is becoming increasingly common among AN patients as a means of relieving their mental suffering.

12.1 Phenomenology

Although the objective psychopathology is similar, the core experiences (phenomenology) of AN and BN patients are different. Both accord an unduly high salience to weight and shape, are preoccupied with eating and not eating, relate low self-esteem to their view of their own bodies, and tend either to deny their thinness or to overestimate their size, but none of these features is unique to these illnesses. Obese girls, binge eaters, and even many healthy young women have similar cognitions. What distinguishes BN and AN patients is the intensity of the cognitions. However, in BN, these concerns are the essence of the disorder. The BN patient seeks slenderness but wants it in order to be healthy and happy. It may be foolish, but it is not irrational. In AN, this is true only in the early phase of the disease. AN patients come to believe that they are not worthy of life, that they do not deserve any form of gratification, that they must punish themselves by unrelenting exercise, that they are not like other people, and that what is acceptable in others is not acceptable in them. If they let up on their anorexic behaviors, then they are filled with self-loathing and guilt. Being emaciated is a goal in itself, not a means of achieving happiness. Work is an obsession, driven by fear of failure rather than by hope of success. It is not that they are closed to reason about their physical condition, but rather that it is irrelevant because the sole purpose of their lives is their abstinence. The extent of their divorce from the reality that most of us recognize may be so great that they are incapable of being responsible for their decisions in relation to their illness.

Do dieting disorder patients have more dysfunctional cognitions and cognitive styles than the non-clinical population? Current data support a cognitive model of dieting disorders. Patients exhibit a lack of awareness of the role played by inner sensations in regulating weight and eating behavior, emphasizing black and white rules instead. Anorexic patients tend to evaluate self-worth almost entirely in terms of self-control. Both patient groups evidence extreme negativity in their views of themselves, but anorexics show a particularly severe sense of self-isolation. Unlike bulimics, they extend a tendency to think in absolute terms from the area of eating to the rest of their lives. Thus, the psychopathology of the anorexic patient group appears more severe than that of bulimics. The basis of BN patients' sense of difference appears to be grounded at least partly in their feelings about weight. If weight were equalized, then they see themselves as fairly similar to others. Anorexics do not follow this pattern: they rate themselves differently to all others, regardless of their own or another's weight.

A key feature of AN is deliberate loss of weight, which is achieved by strict dieting and the avoidance of foods that are perceived to be fattening. Starvation continues despite excessive hunger and cravings for food, and subsequently leads to confused perceptions regarding physiological signals of hunger, so that sufferers may lose the ability to know when they are hungry.

In addition to the avoidance of "fattening" foods, various weight-loss tactics may also be employed.

Another key feature of AN is the excessive concern about weight, shape, eating, and fear of weight gain. This concern persists as an intrusive, overvalued idea. (An overvalued idea is one that is held firmly and that is extremely difficult, although not impossible, to shake.) Concerns about shape and weight have an exaggerated influence on self-image in general. Such concerns produce marked distress and dysfunction among people with dieting disorders. Consequently, they set very low and unrealistic target weights for themselves and do not acknowledge that they have a problem with their weight or eating behaviors, at least early on in their illness. Later on, they may acknowledge that they have problems in these areas but they feel helpless about changing their fears or behaviors. Typically, they have low self-esteem and obsessional traits.

12.2 How is anorexia nervosa different from normal dieting?

- Weight-loss goals are unreasonably low for the person's shape and frame and are changing constantly, so that once a weight-loss goal has been attained, a new, lower goal is set.
- The dieting behavior is solitary. Most "normal" dieters discuss their dieting progress and tactics with their peers. Determined, solitary dieting should be regarded warily.
- The patient is usually dissatisfied with success. Most dieters are pleased if they lose a few kilograms. Successful dieters who remain self-critical may be at risk.

Chapter 13
Specific psychological therapies

13.1 Anorexia nervosa

The few published controlled outcome studies in AN are plagued by problems, including small sample size, contamination of the independent variable through unequal numbers of therapists in each group, the control group having a different therapist to the treatment group, and the investigator also acting as therapist. In some studies, the intervention of interest has been delivered as part of a multimodal package, and it is unclear as to what extent outcome was related to the treatment ingredient. Despite these limitations, it is possible to identify common themes in the psychological approaches to AN and some therapeutic strategies that are potentially valuable.

Cognitive behavioral therapy in anorexia nervosa

In cognitive behavioral therapy (CBT), there is explicit emphasis on beliefs, assumptions, schematic processing, and meaning systems as mediating variables to account for maladaptive emotions and behaviors. CBT sees the central phenomenon of AN as the set of beliefs, attitudes, and assumptions about the meaning of body weight. Thinness is held as the principal construct on which self-worth is based. The anorexic eating behavior is also maintained by a series of negative (avoidance of developmental challenges of puberty, avoidance of performance expectations, avoidance of puberty) and positive (perceptions of control, positive comments from others, feelings of achievement and self-efficacy) reinforcers. The combination of positive and negative reinforcement that maintains the AN helps to explain the egosyntonic nature of the illness.

Treatment has three phases. The first phase includes assessing and addressing the egosyntonic nature of the illness, increasing motivation for change, and developing a formulation of the function of the anorexia for the individual. Target weights and prescribed eating patterns are set. The second phase involves challenging the dysfunctional beliefs about food, eating, and weight, as well as deficits in self-concept. Hence, the cognitive behavioral approach sees weight normalization as a core, but not necessarily sufficient, goal of treatment. Therapy also attempts to modify the meanings attributed to weight and shape, as well as to expand the patient's self-concept from a basis in appearance to a more comprehensive experience of self. The third and final stage of therapy focuses on increasing the patient's awareness of potential triggers for relapse and taking preventive action.

Second, a completely different CBT approach has been proposed, namely that cognitive therapy should focus on the excessive need for self-control through control over weight and shape. An excessive need for self-control plays a role in the onset and maintenance of the AN, as dietary restriction enhances initial feelings of being in control but eventually leads to the physiological and psychological changes, such as intense hunger or hypervigilance to weight or shape changes, that undermine the individual's sense of control and result in an increased effort to control dietary intake. Cognitive therapy targets the use of eating, shape, and weight as indices of self-control and self-worth and the need for excessive self-control in general.

Very few controlled treatment outcome studies have specifically evaluated CBT in AN. One group compared treatment effectiveness of individual CBT, behavior therapy, and an "eclectic" treatment. There were no significant differences between any of the groups on any outcome measure, except that the CBT group had a lower drop-out rate. At the end of treatment, no group was considered to be doing well. A second group of researchers randomly allocated 35 patients with AN to either CBT or dietary advice conditions. At the end of treatment, no group was considered to be doing well. At six months, CBT patients showed significant improvement in BMI. Another study used a modified version of CBT for BN in a case series of five outpatients with AN. Only two of these patients, notably those with purging symptoms, were reported to show improvement. A number of unpublished, randomized, controlled trials of CBT provide some additional evidence regarding the efficacy of this therapy. Ball compared the outcome of individual CBT with that of behavioral family therapy (BFT). Results indicated that both treatment groups showed significant improvement in nutritional status, eating attitudes and behaviors, perfectionism, and self-esteem. However, scores in both treatment conditions remained in the symptomatic range for eating behaviors and attitudes, self-esteem, and depression.

Family therapy

Family therapy in AN is based on the premise that a change in the family system will result in a reduction in the eating disordered behavior. The structural model focuses on the family's way of relating, rather than on just the individual with AN. Based on clinical observations, five characteristics typical of families of individuals with AN were identified. These included enmeshment, rigidity, overprotection, poor conflict resolution, and the involvement of the anorexic individual in unresolved parental conflict. The strategic model proposes that the anorexic individual serves a homeostatic and stabilizing role in the family. Families presenting with an anorexic child were considered to be characterized by a high degree of rigidity, marital dysfunction, poor communication, poor conflict resolution, and a tendency to blame each other. Families were seen to form coalitions and displayed poor boundaries separating the generations in the family.

Cognitive behavioral models of family therapy focus on the ineffective communication of cognitive and emotional messages in the family and emphasize the importance of individuals' assumptions and interpretations of family functioning.

There have been no systematic examinations of the effectiveness of any of these treatments.

The Maudsley group compared the efficacy of family therapy and supportive individual therapy over 12 months in treating AN. The initial focus of family therapy was to gain and maintain family cooperation and then to assess family organization. The most common family intervention was emphasizing and facilitating parental cooperation, mutual support, consistency, and resoluteness. This study involved 57 patients with AN following a period of inpatient weight restoration. Family therapy was more effective in preventing relapse amongst younger patients with disease of early onset (under 19 years of age at onset of illness) and short duration (less than three years), while individual therapy was more effective in older patients.

Another study compared behavioral family systems therapy (BFST) with ego-oriented individual therapy (EOIT) in 22 young adolescents with a short history of AN. BFST focused on encouraging parents to take control of their child's eating and weight gain. EOIT consisted of cognitive interventions around issues such as adolescent autonomy. Both treatments produced significant gains in BMI, eating attitudes, and body satisfaction.

Finally, an Australian study comparing individual CBT and BFT is of note here. In this study, BFT consisted of psycho-education, teaching parental management of eating behaviors, and enhancing communication and problem-solving in the family. Scores for anorexics in both treatment conditions remained in the symptomatic range for eating behaviors and attitudes, self-esteem, and depression.

There is now a widely held assumption, based largely on the work of the Maudsley group, that family therapy is the most effective form of therapy for adolescent patients with a short history of anorexia. Notably, the family interventions that were useful were non-blaming and emphasized the family's responsibility in finding solutions for improving their child's eating behaviors.

Feminist therapy

While there is considerable diversity in feminist thought, feminist understandings of eating disorders hold that cultural constructions of gender are central to eating disorders and are viewed as natural responses to pathological social pressures to be thin rather than being indicative of overt psychopathology. Feminist therapy therefore aims to assist women to examine their behavior in the light of an extreme but not surprising reaction to a gendered and pathological social structure and environment. Two interrelated cultural factors that draw particular attention in feminist approaches are the cultural disempowerment of women and the pressure to attain an unrealistically thin, culturally imposed beauty ideal. Therapy, therefore, is directed towards empowerment of the patient so that they may take control of their life in a less self-destructive manner. The greater the internalization of the thin ideal stereotype, the more frequent the presence of risk factors for AN; particular subcultural environments, such as environments in which peer and family weight concerns are high, are associated with the greater presence of risk factors for eating disorder. Feminist therapies aim to address these cultural pressures.

As a developing approach to therapeutic intervention for AN, feminist orientations have yet to be evaluated empirically.

Combined therapy

An early study compared 12 sessions of combined psychodynamic outpatient therapy and family therapy with 12 sessions of dietary advice. One year after treatment, both groups showed improvements in weight. However, only the dietary advice groups showed a statistically significant weight gain. Social and sexual adjustment were more improved for the psychotherapy–family therapy group. The Maudsley group had used a supportive, educational, and problem-oriented individual therapy and compared it with family therapy. Therapy followed an inpatient weight-restoration program. The individual supportive psychotherapy was found to be effective for patients who were older than 19 years. In a five-year follow-up, these patients continued to gain weight after completing therapy.

Another Maudsley group treated 30 older patients with AN as outpatients with cognitive analytical therapy (CAT), which integrates psychodynamic and behavioral factors and focuses on interpersonal and transference issues. This form of therapy was compared with an educational behavioral treatment. Strong overall outcomes were obtained by the study, with 63% of the clients being within 15% of normal body weight (good outcome) and having normal menstrual cycles at one year post-treatment. The group given CAT reported significantly greater subjective improvement, but there were no differences in other outcome parameters between the treatment groups.

Given the evidence reviewed above, moderate confidence may be placed in therapies that combine cognitive and psychodynamic strategies.

Motivational therapy

The goal of motivational interviewing is to facilitate the patient's readiness to change. Motivational enhancement therapy targets the egosyntonic nature of the illness, which has been defined as the "potent positive sense of self-reinforcement anorexics seem to obtain from their symptoms." While using strategies to enhance motivation to change is intuitively compelling in a psychological treatment of AN, it should be noted that there is no published empirical evidence supporting their use.

Interpersonal psychotherapy

Interpersonal factors have been prominent in the etiological models of AN, and the presence of difficulties in interpersonal functioning among anorexic patients has received empirical support. Interpersonal psychotherapy (IPT) was developed originally as a manualized psychotherapy for depression. A modified form was used to act as a control group in a randomized control trial for CBT for BN. IPT posits that although people may experience various pathways into the eating disorder, interpersonal difficulties contribute to the onset and maintenance of the condition. IPT is described as a present-oriented, non-interpretative, individual psychotherapy with a focus on linking current interpersonal problems and interpersonal functioning to eating problems. In the manualized version of IPT for BN, the eating disorder symptoms per se are explicitly never directly the focus of sessions. Not discussing the core presenting symptom is a departure from the

IPT manuals for depression, which advocate continual evaluation of depressive symptomatology. In AN, it is recommended not only that IPT includes a continual review of the links between core anorexic symptoms and the interpersonal problem area of interest, but that neglecting these potentially life-threatening features of anorexia is undesirable and unethical. Critically low body weight may be a contraindication for IPT, and continued weight loss during IPT might necessitate a suspension of IPT towards more supportive interventions while physical state is stabilised. A New Zealand trial compared IPT, CBT, and simple supportive therapy in preventing relapse in AN patients. Simple supportive therapy appeared the most efficacious.

Evidence-based therapy

There is evidence to suggest that some treatment of a general nature for AN results in lower mortality than no treatment at all and is therefore to be recommended. Family-based approaches have moderate support as effective treatments for AN, especially in younger patients who have a short history of the disorder. Individual CBT also has moderate support as an effective treatment for AN. Combined treatments, especially an integration of psychodynamic and cognitive behavioral treatments, but also family and psychodynamic therapies, have moderate support as effective treatments. Under any system, it is important that the therapist respects, and does not flout, the patient's set of values, while at the same time not condoning the illness.

Guidelines based on theoretical frameworks
- Establishment of a sound therapeutic relationship.
- Enhancement of motivation for change.
- Restoration of a normal body weight.
- Provision of strategies to cope with nutritional restoration.
- Modification of abnormal attitudes about eating, weight, and shape.
- Restoration of more normal interpersonal functioning and developing more adaptive coping strategies.
- Modification of deficits in self-concept and self-esteem.
- Management of issues of personal effectiveness, control, and power.

Evidence-based medicine in anorexia nervosa
Despite general consensus about acute treatment, there is little evidence-based literature to support current practices. Some, such as the reversal of serious medical complications, appear obvious. Others are perhaps less easy to support.

Among the issues that require scientific study are the following:

- Is it better to restore nutritional state rapidly (e.g. by nasogastric tube feeding) and then normalize eating behavior? Or should one seek to normalize nutrition by normalizing eating from the start?
- Is rapid refeeding preferable to, or less valuable than, gradual refeeding?
- Is it necessary to restore the patient to a normal state of nutrition while in acute treatment, or merely to get them back to a safe weight? And if the former, is normal nutrition rightly assessed as being within the normal weight range, or does it mean a return to premorbid weight?
- Anorexia patients selectively avoid high-energy, fatty foods. Should weight restoration on a predominantly carbohydrate diet be condoned, or should the patient be pushed to include normal proportions of fats and proteins?
- Hypothermia, if pronounced, must be treated. But is there a place for warming all patients so that they maintain a normal core body temperature?
- Do psychotropic drugs exert any beneficial effect on the course of AN? Are they effective against the secondary psychiatric symptoms, e.g. are antidepressants effective against depressive symptoms in the context of the illness or against obsessive-compulsive symptoms? (There have been no trials directed at this specific issue.)
- Is psychotherapy beneficial? And if so, is there anything specific about the psychotherapy, or is it simply the support it provides? Cognitive therapy is generally chosen, but is there evidence that it actually works in anorexia (as it does in BN)? What about insight-oriented or interpersonal psychotherapy or family therapy?

It is deplorable that so many relatively simple questions relating to the treatment of AN have not yet been subjected to experimental study. The few facts that have emerged are the following:

- Lenient and flexible behavioral programs are no less effective than strict approaches.
- Frequency of weighing does not appear to have an influence, and short-term behavioral programs are usually perceived by patients as helpful, albeit boring.
- Family therapy is preferable to individual psychotherapy in patients.

13.2 Bulimia nervosa

The relative paucity of research on outcomes of treatment for AN contrasts sharply with the quantity and quality of research on outcomes of treatment for BN. Effective treatment is available in the form of CBT, IPT, nutritional counseling, and the use of antidepressant drugs, particularly SSRIs. There is a solid foundation of evidence-based research.

Specially trained and interested psychologists and dietitians usually provide non-pharmacological treatment. However, psychologists, psychiatrists, and dietitians are often available only in large, urban centres, and then only by private payment. Thus, although effective treatment is available, many people with BN or BED cannot afford to access it.

Admission to hospital is rarely required; when it does occur, it is usually because of safety concerns in relation to the risk of suicide. Depression is a prominent feature associated with BN and BED and needs to be considered in planning treatment. Prevention strategies would seem to be indicated because of the demonstrated relationship of these syndromes to the "thinness ideal," complementing early identification and intervention, but so far they have proved disappointing.

Pharmacotherapy

A large number of good to excellent outcome studies suggest that several different classes of antidepressant drugs produce significantly greater reductions in the short term for binge eating and purging in BN patients than a placebo treatment. The long-term effects of antidepressant medication on BN remain untested.

Several conclusions can be drawn from the antidepressant drug studies to date:

- Most antidepressant drugs are more effective than a pill placebo for reducing binge eating and purging.
- With one exception, there have been no systematic dose–response studies. The exception showed that 60 mg/day, but not 20 mg/day, of fluoxetine is more effective than a pill placebo. There is no correlation between tricyclic serum levels and response.
- Different classes of antidepressants seem to be equally effective. However, there have been no direct comparisons of different drugs within the same study. At present, fluoxetine (60 mg daily) would appear to be the drug of choice because of its relative freedom from adverse side effects.
- Patients who fail to respond to an initial antidepressant drug may respond to another.
- The long-term effects of antidepressant medication remain largely untested.
- Few drug studies have evaluated the effects of antidepressant medication on aspects of BN other than binge eating and purging.

- Consistent predictors of a positive response to antidepressant medication have yet to be identified.
- The mechanisms by which antidepressant medication exerts its effects are unknown. Its effects cannot be mediated by reductions in depression since pretreatment levels of depression are unrelated to outcome. The apparent comparability of different classes of antidepressant drugs suggests some mechanism common to these agents. One possibility is that antidepressant medication attenuates hunger, thereby making it easier for BN patients to maintain their strict dieting. There is evidence that fluoxetine produces a small but significant short-term reduction in weight in BN patients.

Cognitive behavioral therapy

A very substantial number of well-designed studies have shown that manual-based CBT is currently the first-line treatment of choice for BN; roughly half of patients receiving CBT cease binge eating and purging. Well-accepted by patients, CBT is the most effective means of eliminating the characteristic behavioral features and is often accompanied by improvement in comorbid psychological problems, such as low self-esteem and depression. Long-term maintenance of improvement is reasonably good.

CBT for BN is based on a model that emphasizes the critical role of both cognitive and behavioral factors in the maintenance of the disorder.

Of primary importance is the extreme personal value that is attached to an idealized body shape and low body weight. This results in an extreme and rigid restriction of food intake, which in turn makes patients physiologically and psychologically susceptible to periodic episodes of loss of control over eating (i.e. binge eating). The episodes are, in part, maintained by negative reinforcement, since they temporarily reduce negative affect. Purging and other extreme forms of weight control are used in an attempt to compensate for the effects on weight of binge eating. Purging reinforces binge eating by temporarily reducing the anxiety about potential weight gain and by disrupting the learned satiety that regulates food intake. In turn, binge eating and purging cause distress and lower self-esteem, thereby reciprocally fostering the conditions that will inevitably lead to more dietary restraint and binge eating.

Treatment must address more than the presenting behaviors of binge eating and purging. The extreme dietary restraint must be replaced with a more normal pattern of eating, and the dysfunctional thoughts and attitudes about body shape and weight must also be addressed.

The treatment is conducted on an outpatient basis and is suitable for all patients, apart from the small minority (less than 5%) who require hospitalization. A detailed manual is available.

A summary in 1991 of ten studies yielded a mean reduction in purging of 79%, with a 57% remission figure. A tally of nine controlled studies of CBT published after this review yields estimates of a mean reduction in purging of 83.5%, with a 47.5% remission figure. The comparable estimates for binge eating are 79% and 62%, respectively.

Main elements of cognitive behavioral therapy for bulimia nervosa

* Good therapeutic relationship.
* Self-monitoring.
* Education about the cognitive model.
* Regular weekly weighing.
* Education about body weight regulation, the adverse effects of dieting, and the consequences of purging.
* Regular pattern of eating (three meals a day plus planned snacks).
* Self-control strategies (e.g. stimulus control techniques).
* Problem-solving.
* Modifying rigid dieting.
* Cognitive restructuring for overcoming concerns about eating and body shape and weight.
* Exposure methods for increasing acceptance of body.
* Relapse-prevention training.

CBT has been shown to be consistently superior to wait-list control groups. A more powerful approach to evaluating CBT is to compare its effects directly with alternative treatments within the same study. Comparisons of CBT and antidepressant drugs suggest the following conclusions:

* CBT seems more acceptable to patients than antidepressant medication.
* The drop-out rate is lower with CBT than with pharmacological treatments.
* CBT seems to be superior to treatment with a single antidepressant drug.
* Combining CBT with antidepressant medication is significantly more effective than using medication alone.
* Combining CBT and antidepressant medication produces few consistent benefits over CBT alone.
* Longer-term maintenance of change appears to be better with CBT than with antidepressant drugs.

Recently, CBT has been shown to be effective in a group setting as well as in individual therapy setting.

Focal interpersonal psychotherapy

CBT has been compared with an adaptation of a form of brief focal psychotherapy. The rationale for the latter treatment is that BN is maintained by a variety of ongoing problems (mostly of an interpersonal nature), and that to overcome the eating disorder these problems have to be identified and resolved. The focal psychotherapy included the self-monitoring of binge eating, since binges are often triggered by interpersonal problems, and therefore they can serve as a useful marker of such problems. Both treatments produced striking improvements in the core symptomatology of BN at post-treatment and over a one-year closed follow-up.

A second study from the same group is also one of the best controlled studies to date. CBT was compared with two alternative treatments. The first was behavior therapy, comprising the CBT treatment minus cognitive restructuring and the behavioral and cognitive methods for modifying abnormal attitudes about weight and shape; the second treatment was an adaptation of IPT. In the latter treatment, little attention was paid to the eating disorder per se. All three treatments were manual-based, and their implementation was monitored closely. The Eating Disorder Examination (EDE) was used as the main measure of outcome.

At post-treatment, the three therapies were equally effective in reducing binge eating. The mean reductions were 71% for CBT, 62% for behavioral therapy, and 62% for IPT. However, CBT was significantly more effective than IPT in reducing purging, dietary restraint, and attitudes to shape and weight, and superior to behavioral therapy on the last two variables despite equivalent ratings of suitability of treatment and expectations of outcome. This pattern of results shows that CBT had specific effects on different measures of outcome consistent with its theoretical rationale. As in the previous study by the Oxford group, treatment was followed by a one-year closed follow-up (i.e. it was treatment-free). This showed that the effects of CBT were well maintained and significantly superior to behavioral therapy but equal to IPT. The patients were followed up once more after an average of 5.8 (SD ± 2.0) years, thereby providing a unique perspective of the long-term impact of these three treatments. There was a clear difference among them: those patients who had received CBT or IPT were doing equally well, with 63% and 72% respectively, having no DSM-IV eating disorder, compared with 14% for those who had received behavioral therapy.

Behavioral therapy

A collaborative Australian-German study compared a nutritional management treatment with stress management. The former closely approximated the behavioral components of CBT; the latter included standard cognitive behavioral strategies, such as active coping and problem-solving, but never focused directly on the modification of eating or attitudes about weight and shape. The results showed marginally significant but consistent differences in favor of nutritional management both at post-treatment and at one-year follow-up. Nutritional management produced significantly more rapid changes in eating behavior and purging than stress management.

A related study compared intensive nutritional counseling combined with either fluoxetine (60 mg) or pill placebo for eight weeks of individual treatment. The nutritional counseling used by this Australian group was a form of psychoeducational treatment that focused on correcting misconceptions about eating and body weight, and on replacing unhealthy dieting with normal eating. It shared some of the educational and behavioral features of CBT, such as self-monitoring and self-control techniques (e.g. stimulus control), but it lacked the systematic cognitive focus and techniques of CBT. The two treatments showed equivalent, clinically significant reductions in binge eating and purging at the end of eight weeks. The only advantage for the active drug was on the restraint and shape and weight concern subscales of the EDE. A three-month follow-up showed that the improvement in binge eating and purging was maintained, but that the fluoxetine was no longer superior to pill placebo on the EDE subscales.

Psychodynamic psychotherapy

Controlled studies of the effectiveness of psychodynamic therapies are lacking. Despite the absence of data to support the use of psychodynamic psychotherapy for the treatment of BN, this therapy remains very popular in the USA.

Family therapy

The American Psychiatric Association's practice guidelines assert that family-oriented therapies may be especially useful in the treatment of BN, yet only a single controlled study has evaluated the effectiveness of a family therapy approach. This study was marked by a high drop-out rate (44%) and an unusually poor outcome.

Conclusions

- Manual-based CBT is currently the treatment of choice for BN.
- CBT is superior to behavioral versions of the treatment that omit cognitive restructuring and the focus is on modifying attitudes toward body shape and weight.
- CBT is significantly more effective than, or at least as effective as, any form of psychotherapy with which it has been compared.
- CBT produces a clinically significant degree of improvement.
- CBT reliably produces changes across all four of the specific features of BN, namely binge eating, purging, dietary restraint, and abnormal attitudes about body shape and weight.
- CBT is comparatively fast-acting.
- CBT affects both the specific and general psychopathology of BN.
- CBT is associated with good maintenance of change at six-months and one-year follow-up.
- No reliable predictors of response to CBT have been identified.

CBT was designed for use within specialist settings. It is time-consuming (involving about 20 sessions over five months) and, to be executed optimally, training is required. There is a need to develop simpler and briefer forms of CBT suitable for widespread use.

Not every patient requires the full program of individual CBT. Some patients respond to briefer and simpler interventions, including cognitive behavioral self-help manuals, brief group psychoeducational programs, versions of CBT designed for use by non-specialists in primary care, and CBT delivered in a group. The chief limitation of CBT is that a significant proportion of patients do not make a full response. Different options for improving on the success rate of CBT have been elaborated. One strategy would be to combine CBT with antidepressant medication, but there is little evidence that combining CBT with antidepressant medication significantly enhances improvement.

13.3 Binge eating disorder

BED is characterized by recurrent episodes of binge eating in the absence of the extreme methods of weight control seen in BN. Thus, there is no purging, overexercising, or extreme and rigid dieting. Rather, the binge eating occurs against a background of a general tendency to overeat. Not surprisingly, many patients with BED are overweight or frankly obese. The disorder is accompanied by concerns about shape and weight, but these are more understandable than those seen in BN given these patients' weight. Unlike in BN, self-evaluation tends not to be focused on shape and weight. Partly for this reason, the relevance to BED of the cognitive model of BN has been questioned. Like BN, however, BED is associated with shame and self-recrimination and some degree of psychosocial impairment.

While controlled studies of their long-term effectiveness are lacking, several different psychological treatments appear equally effective in reducing the frequency of binge eating in the short term in BED. These treatments include CBT, interpersonal therapy, and behavioral weight loss programs, with or without an accompanying very-low-calorie diet (VLCD). There is currently little evidence that antidepressant medication is effective for treating binge eating in BED patients.

In BED, the aim of treatment is to establish healthy eating habits by helping patients avoid all forms of overeating. As in BN, the successful resolution of the eating disorder is generally associated with a marked decrease in associated psychosocial impairment.

The first point that must be emphasized is that the research on the treatment of BED is at an early stage. As mentioned above, the histories of these patients suggest that, unlike BN, it is a phasic condition with extended periods of remission. The disorder also appears vulnerable to "placebo effects," in that substantial improvement often occurs among those allocated to delayed treatment control conditions or a pill placebo. Contrary to some suggestions, it has emerged that treatments that encourage dietary restraint do not promote binge eating among those with BED.

There are too few pharmacotherapy studies to draw firm conclusions about the use of drugs for the treatment of BED. Nevertheless, it should be noted that four of the five controlled studies of antidepressant medication showed no advantage of the drug over a placebo. This finding is very different from that for BN.

Overall, the results to date reinforce the differences between BED and BN.

PART V

Areas of special interest

Introduction

This section of the book is directed at a more selective audience than Parts I–IV. First, it deals with the specific roles that general practitioners, nurses, and dietitians play in the management of patients with AN and other eating disorders. Second, it provides a brief section on the essential information that should be given to patients, their families, and their friends. Third, it draws conclusions about the possible future direction of clinical work in eating disorders and to the possibility of prevention programs with an appraisal of risk factors.

Chapter 14

The role of the general practitioner

With the current shift in focus from tertiary services to primary and secondary services, and with estimates that up to 5% of women presenting to (or registered with) a general practitioner have an eating disorder, the general practitioner's (GP) role in identifying, treating, and managing people with eating disorders is becoming increasingly important. In addition, it is particularly concerning that, because eating disorders are frequently concealed or denied, up to 50% of cases go unrecognized in a clinical setting. On a practical level, secondary prevention has been associated with improved outcome and reduced chronicity.

For patients with partial- and full-syndrome disorders, the most effective role that a GP can take is the role of care coordinator or case manager. As Keks notes, "There is no consensus as to what constitutes case management; [however] on an individual patient level it means the coordination of care for patients who require a number of services from different providers."

In some cases, the GP's main goal will be to build rapport and motivation for change before arranging referral to other health professionals for treatment. In other instances, where additional training has been undertaken, the GP may feel comfortable with taking on an extended role. Alternatively, the GP may wish to limit actual practice to medical management but to take responsibility for coordinating associated services. An essential component of every GP's role is the identification of the disorder as it presents in various developmental or formative stages.

First, GPs are asked to identify those patients at risk of developing eating disorders (the extreme dieter) and to implement appropriate early intervention or risk-reduction strategies. Second, GPs should detect and monitor those with partial-syndrome disorders (EDNOS), developing a rapport with the patient, and encouraging them to normalize eating and behavior patterns in an attempt to prevent the development of a full-syndrome disorder. Third, GPs must diagnose those patients with full-syndrome eating disorders (AN), engage them in treatment, monitor their progress and medical condition, and provide consistent and continuous care across the treatment spectrum and across the illness trajectory.

However, identifying patients with eating disorders, and those at risk of developing eating disorders, is not as simple as it may first appear. Turnbull found that in primary practice, the median time between the onset and diagnosis of AN was approximately one year.

Noordenbos highlighted the various problems that may prevent the GP from timely identification of eating disorders. The first subset of problems she calls "patient delay." This includes those instances where the patient denies that they have eating disorder or engages surreptitiously in the disordered behaviors. Vandereycken and Meerman state that, at times, families may also unwittingly collude with the patient in hiding the disorder. However, ultimately 90% of eating disorder patients present to their GP with associated complaints, frequently hoping that the doctor will pick up on a small hint and probe further about dieting behavior. The failure to pick up on such "hints" is a marker of a second subset of problems ("doctor delay").

A particular problem for GPs is the difficulty in identifying the early signs of eating disorders when not all diagnostic criteria are met. Doctor delay may also be associated with negative attitudes about the perceived self-inflicted nature of the eating disorders. The GP's interest, skill, and ability in psychiatry in general, and in eating disorders in particular, will also impact on illness detection, as will the GP's ability to accept that a young, intelligent, active teenager can be gravely ill.

A set of structural difficulties also exists and will be encountered by GPs, potentially impeding their ability to effectively manage eating disorder patients. These include the amount of time available and required to care for patients with eating disorders and appropriate remuneration for this time.

There are a number of advantages associated with GPs acting as the primary care coordinator. First, GPs offer affordable access to comprehensive care that can be accessed widely and relatively rapidly. Second, there is no stigma attached to consulting a GP. Third, patients with eating disorders are known to attend GPs more frequently in the five years before diagnosis than other patients. Fourth, GPs are usually familiar with the patient and the family involved, and as such can provide much needed support and advice during episodes of illness as well as an holistic understanding of the family and its members. And fifth, GPs are well placed to manage those with chronic conditions such as AN.

Eating disorder patients are most likely to present to GPs with eating or weight concerns, providing evidence that a higher index of suspicion is warranted for some demographic groups. Females with AN present to GPs at a rate of 34.1 per 100 000 in the 10–19 years age range, and patients with BN present at a rate of 56.7 per 100 000 in women aged 20–39 years.

GPs should maintain a high index of suspicion when women aged between ten and 40 years present with gynecological complaints (most commonly amenorrhea or irregular menses), gastrointestinal problems, (including nausea, unexplained vomiting, constipation, food "allergies"), psychological symptoms (depressed mood, insomnia, increasing anxiety), and overt concern about body weight or shape (requests for diet pills, a special diet, actual weight loss).

Screening should entail:

- knowledge of family members and their relationships;
- regular recording of the subject's weight and height;
- enquiry about general health and wellbeing;
- menstruation;
- nutritional intake;
- physical activity;
- involvement in elite sports;
- involvement in high-risk occupations or activities.

Poorer prognoses in both AN and BN are associated with low weight at presentation, a history of failure to respond to treatment, disturbed family relationships, and personality disorder. In addition, patients with AN and who vomit, and those with BN and who purge, have a poorer prognosis. The factors said to contribute to an eating disorder becoming chronic include unresolved family and interpersonal issues and an inability to give up the anorexic stance.

Nutritional rehabilitation and weight gain are important early goals in the treatment of AN (and also in subclinical presentations and extreme dieting); they are necessary for psychological treatments or medical interventions to be effective.

Where a GP elects to take on the management of a patient with AN, the GP will be responsible for setting acceptable goals and limits for the patient's nutritional status and weight.

Where a GP does not elect to take on the management of a patient with AN, but they have identified the disease in their patient, the GP is obliged to confer with and refer the patient to an experienced dietitian.

- Accelerated weight loss of more than 1 kg/week is an indication for inpatient admission.
- Monitor weight regularly.

- Inability to gain weight as an outpatient or insidious weight loss over time indicates that the patient needs additional specialist treatment.
- The goal for all patients is to reach their target weight range.
- A realistic compromise may be necessary for patients with chronic AN – 40% of cases do not recover fully.
- In adults with chronic AN, a BMI of 16 or more is associated with short-term medical stability if weight remains constant. A BMI of 13 or less is associated with increased medical complications, therefore a medical admission should be considered.

The indications for referral to a specialist service are as follows:

- BMI falls below 16;
- unremitting weight loss;
- abnormal EKG, with QTc greater than 450 ms, abnormal pacemaker, or ventricular dysrhythmia;
- deficiency of potassium, magnesium or phosphorus;
- decreased serum albumen;
- volume depletion or azotemia;
- temperature of less than 36 °C;
- unsuccessful outpatient treatment after three months of active treatment.

Most GPs will easily determine the point at which their patients require admission. The signs specific to AN indicating a need for hospitalization include:

- BMI falls below 13;
- symptomatic dysrhythmia;
- abnormal biochemistry: electrolyte disturbance;
- presyncope or syncope due to hypoglycemia, hypotension, or dysrhythmia;
- metabolic complications secondary to purging behavior;
- patient is suicidal;
- special considerations:
  - diabetes (where the risk of blindness and kidney damage is increased);
  - pregnancy after 24 weeks.

14.1 Chronic anorexia nervosa

- Treatment of concurrent medical and psychiatric conditions is always indicated.
- The treatment of malnutrition is limited only by a risk–benefit trade-off.

- Focus on improved quality of life through rehabilitation.
- Finally, remember that AN may remit at any time in its course.

Clinical remission in chronic AN usually occurs due to sociological change (e.g. divorce, death of a parent, decision to change careers) or because the patient simply becomes tired of being burdened with AN.

All patients with AN can recover – and some recover decades into their illness. However, while the patient continues to suffer from chronic AN, the important model of treatment is one of rehabilitation.

Patients with chronic AN have ongoing signs and symptoms of protein-calorie malnutrition. They will have thinning of the hair, dry and yellow skin, decreased ability to focus the eyes, shortness of breath on exertion, decreased exercise capacity, repeated dysrhythmias, dizziness on standing, weakness, tiredness, hypothermia, muscle cramps, and decreased memory and concentration. In addition, they will suffer from progressive osteopenia, which will cause repeated fractures; these begin as stress fractures and later become symptomatic fractures of the spine and lower extremities.

Chronic AN is associated with social isolation, an inability to work and learn, and diminished functional activity, including with family and friends and at work. Depending on the level of debilitation, the patient may be reclusive, living in a small apartment and isolated from their family, or they may be a thin patient with significant weight and shape concerns but who is fully integrated into their family, work, and society. Clearly, the rehabilitation goal is to move a patient with AN from the former to the latter situation.

The GP should concentrate first on physical complaints. Patients with chronic AN find it much easier to talk about physical concerns. Treatment of physical problems is easily accepted and appreciated, which increases rapport. Treatment of urinary incontinence (which commonly occurs in chronic AN), careful care of feet and toes, and prevention of osteopenia with calcium and vitamin D supplements should all be considered. Use of the birth control pill to continue menstruation and potentially to increase bone mass should be discussed, as might the use of bisphosphonates to halt bone catabolism.

Psychologically, the focus should be on rehabilitation and quality of life. Any comorbid condition, such as a history of sexual abuse, substance abuse, or depression, should be sought and may require long-term treatment before other psychological gains are possible.

One must be very careful regarding the involvement of the family in the treatment of chronic AN. Any discussions with family members are best done at the patient's request and with the patient present.

The use of exercise in chronic AN has been controversial. However, our work in the use of yoga in hospital and with a graded exercise program out of hospital to focus on breathing, stretching, and gradual incorporation of exercise to try to increase lean body mass and maintain bony mass is gaining acceptance. Paradoxically, overexercise may decrease with a graded introduction of minimal activity in the patient with chronic AN. Simply prohibiting activity is unlikely to be accepted by the patient.

The GP should refer patients with chronic AN for specific physical complaints such as osteoporosis.

Chapter 15

Nursing patients with anorexia nervosa

15.1 Introduction

Caring for patients with dieting disorders can be one of the most challenging and rewarding roles for nurses. However, even for the most experienced clinician, it can also be frustrating, anxiety-provoking, and emotionally draining, and nurses must be aware of the potential for burnout and emotional over- or underinvolvement.

Nurses become many things to a patient with AN, most essentially someone who is familiar with the patient's feelings, ideas, emotions, routines, rituals, and behaviors. Nurses need to be skilled in recognizing and interpreting the physiological and psychological signs, symptoms, and complications of the disorder. It is imperative that they develop an empathic, non-judgmental approach, and that they maintain clear professional boundaries – yet a nurse's job is to challenge fixed and unrealistic beliefs and to assist in the development of motivation to change, so it is necessary to form a strong and trusting bond. As well, nurses provide information, act as role models, and support the patient and their family through the recovery process.

In order to fulfill this challenging and difficult role, nurses need education, clinical supervision, support from management and administration, collaboration and communication with other nursing colleagues, and recognition from other members of the treatment team that the nurse's role is valuable and vital.

15.2 The role of the nurse

The role of the nurse in managing patients with AN is varied, and includes the following:

- *Development of rapport between the patient and the treatment team.* In order to promote trust between the patient and the treatment team, the nurse must

245

first develop a therapeutic relationship with the patient. To develop such a relationship, the nurse should become familiar with the patient's thoughts, feelings, and behaviors; understanding the patient's anorexic experience; align with the patient against the disorder; and display an empathic, non-judgmental, but structured approach.

• *Monitoring the patient's physical and mental state.* Because AN combines physiological and psychological complications (which are frequently sequelae of one another), an important function of the nurse's role is to monitor the physical and mental status of the patient. There is a significant risk of death in AN; consequently, nurses must be vigilant for signs and symptoms that may indicate serious or potentially fatal complications. There are several key physiological abnormalities that the nurse must be aware of and recognize – most particularly, the presence of refeeding syndrome, delirium, cardiac complications and renal failure.

The primary metabolic features of the refeeding syndrome are hypophosphatemia, hypokalemia, and hypomagnesemia, and the clinical signs and symptoms include delirium, arrhythmia, cardiac failure or acute myocardial infarction, and sudden death. Nurses caring for patients who are being fed by nasogastric tube must be aware of the physiological processes involved with refeeding and the potential for complications. Routine observations are essential, and distinguishing between the more benign or "usual" pathological signs of AN (bradycardia, hypotension, hypothermia) and the "unusual" pathological signs of refeeding syndrome requires close attention.

Osteoporosis, osteopenia, dehydration, hypothermia, and neurological complications (seizures, peripheral neuritis) are also problematic, as are less severe (but, at times, more disturbing for the patient) problems with constipation, cramps, nausea, dental caries, and enamel erosion. The nurse's role is to monitor the patient's physical status and, where possible, to minimize discomfort, in order that progress is not affected adversely or impeded by the disease sequelae.

The patient's mental state must also be monitored closely. While patients commonly display low or labile mood, poor concentration, disrupted sleep patterns, impaired memory, and obsessive-compulsive features, the nurse should be assessing constantly for signs that may indicate that a secondary diagnosis of major depression or obsessive-compulsive disorder is warranted. As well, the nurse will need to be aware of the cognitive impairments affecting the patient's capacity to absorb new information. Accordingly, psychoeducation and counseling will need to be tailored individually to suit the patient's strengths and weaknesses.

- *Establishing and maintaining a therapeutic milieu and a common philosophical approach.* In the eating disorder unit, specific characteristics of the therapeutic milieu include flexibility within structure and a consensus between staff members regarding the unit's philosophical approach. Although every nurse has a different personality and a different style of nursing, it is important that all staff agree on the overall goals and direction of the program. This enables individual nurses to work flexibly within the program's structure, and reduces the potential for nurses to become bogged down with the procedural details of the program at the expense of the bigger therapeutic picture.
- *Educator, role model, group facilitator, support person, and the voice of reason.* Most patients will have varying levels of understanding of their illness and its direct effect on their thoughts, feelings, and behavior. Nurses should not assume that just because a patient sounds knowledgeable, they are not in need of information – a patient's knowledge might be inaccurate or applied incorrectly.

  Nurses must also take on the important role of working with the patient's family. Through discussion with family members, nurses can gain insight into the patient's strengths and weaknesses, how the patient uses their disorder to communicate, and how the disorder impacts on family dynamics. It will benefit the patient if the nurse can help the family to cope with the illness. Of course, the patient is always the nurse's primary concern, and confidentiality must always be considered. Discussing with the patient the variety of roles that nurses may assume will give the patient the opportunity to ask for the nurse's help and support in family discussions.

  As well as developing and sustaining individual relationships, nurses must act as a group facilitator for all patients in the program. Relationships between patients can deteriorate rapidly, and group dynamics will require close attention from the nurse. Some patients will act as inspiration to others, providing support and a sense of experiential understanding. At other times, patients may vie for the nurse's attention, compete with each other, and undermine one another's self-confidence and the potential of the program to help. It is not uncommon for "good" and "compliant" patients to feel resentful and ignored when a new or very difficult patient absorbs nursing time. The patient may interpret the nurse's distraction as an indication that their problems are less important and/or that the new or difficult patient is sicker or more worthy of attention.

  The nurse's role as the voice of reason is an important one, and its primary feature will be in assisting the patient to broaden their perspective of the disease, their life, and the process of recovery. Assisting the patient to approach recovery from different perspectives, broadening their focus, and reorienting them towards success are all components of this process.

- *Setting limits and maintaining personal and professional boundaries.* Once trust is established, nurses may feel deeply committed to the relationship they have worked so hard to develop. If one considers all the facets of the relationship – friendliness, trust, familiarity, empathy, responsiveness, caring, positive regard – it is easy to see why it could be misconstrued as a friendship, or why one or other of the parties may become confused about the purpose of the relationship. Neither the nurse nor the patient is immune to this confusion. The nurse, particularly if a novice, may become overinvolved with the patient or take personal affront at perceived failures or imposition of limits. It will then be more likely that the nurse experiences problems with counter-transference. The patient may become dependent on the nurse or feel burdened by the confusing messages received from the relationship, and transference may occur.

  For these reasons, it is important that the nurse's roles and responsibilities are defined clearly by the nurse, with the patient, at the start of the relationship. Establishing and maintaining firm boundaries gives the patient and the nurse a focus. If this is not done, it becomes difficult for the nurse to set effective limits – an essential feature supporting the structure of the program.

- *Team coordinator.* Management of patients with eating disorders must be a multidisciplinary effort, and role definition is one of the most important functions involved in the smooth running of the multidisciplinary team.

  The nurse's role includes implementing team management plans and developing nursing management plans where necessary; providing background information required to evaluate the patient's progress by monitoring their dietary intake and level of activity; liaison with the family, the legal guardian, or the mental health tribunal; and supervision of the consistent running of the program. Nurses support and counsel the patient through the difficulties experienced each day and conduct therapeutic groups in tandem with individual programs. Where other members of the treatment team defer to the nurse with regard to day-to-day management of the program (leave, etc.), there are fewer problems with "splitting" between disciplines.

- *Clinical supervision and consistency between nurses.* In order to remain professional, to maintain clear boundaries, and to examine one's personal feelings and emotional responses to the patient's anorexic behavior, clinical supervision and peer support are essential. Nurses should use self-reflection to examine the features of the disease that engender a counter-transference response. Discussing counter-transference issues in a clinical supervision setting will assist the nurse to maintain focus, enthusiasm, and perspective. It will also assist the nurse to maintain the therapeutic alliance.

While it is unlikely that all nurses on a unit will be eager to specialize in eating disorders, they will all need to be aware of the fundamental aspects of the program. This is essential to maintaining consistency with regard to general issues, such as regular periods of bedrest, leave from the unit, and meal routines, and will ensure that nurses are not unnecessarily stringent.

Communication and consistency between staff and team members are vital to the success of a program. Management plans should be documented clearly to avoid problems arising when the primary nurse is off duty, as confusion and lack of consistency cause huge amounts of anxiety for the patient. It is important to remember that consistency does not mean rigidity. A firm but flexible and reasonable approach will improve the likelihood that the patient develops a sense of trust in the primary nurse and the nursing team.

15.3 Conclusion

Nurses are vital members of the eating disorder treatment team. They are skilled in managing the physiological and psychological aspects of the disorders, and they are well placed to making an important impact on the recovery of a hospitalized patient. The nurse's input must be obtained where decisions are being made about policy and service delivery for patients with eating disorders.

Chapter 16

The role of the dietitian

A team approach is vital for effective treatment of eating disorders. The specialist clinical dietitian, as part of the team, is the most qualified person to provide accurate education about nutrition, weight gain, weight maintenance, the resumption of normal eating, and the nutritional methods of avoiding the refeeding syndrome.

Nutrition treatment is not as simple as applying an educational formula and handing out a diet sheet. Nutrition intervention is complex, and eating disorder patients are resistant to nutritional treatment. Compliance may be reduced by perceived coercion, psychiatric comorbidities such as borderline personality disorders, self-harm, and suicidality, and ethical issues such as the need to report at-risk children to the law. Dietary change may be dependent on the patient's psychological progress.

The objectives of this chapter are to:

- Review the range of dietetic interventions that are professionally acceptable to dietitians.
- List some methods of dealing with the emotional issues that are likely to occur during treatment.
- Promote self-care (supervision) for all dietitians working with eating disordered patients.
- Discuss distinctions between specialist and non-specialist dietitians.

16.1 Clinical boundaries

Discuss the therapeutic limitations of nutrition counseling and make clear the need for concurrent psychotherapy at the first interview.

16.2 Professional boundaries

- *Work as a member of a team:* before initiating any nutrition intervention, make certain that a doctor is following the patient medically on a regular basis and that psychological therapy is being carried out by a qualified practitioner. Emphasize the link between the patient's eating disorder and their emotional health in the dietetic sessions. Set an upper limit of six dietetic sessions with a patient who is not engaged in a psychological intervention. This is to avoid clouding the dietetic intervention with emotional issues, to encourage psychological treatment, and to protect the patient against inadequate treatment.
- *How much time should be allowed per dietetic session?* Expect to spend an hour in the first assessment, with up to another hour to discuss your assessment, with the team and debrief. Follow-up sessions may be just as lengthy.
- *How many eating disordered clients is it possible to see in a day?* Expect to be emotionally and physically drained by nutritional work with eating disorder patients. Four or five patients at a contemplative or precontemplative stage of change is sufficient. In the action stage of change, it is possible to see more. Maintain some time free of patient contact to reflect.
- *Discuss the end of treatment at the beginning of treatment:* the average duration of AN is seven years. It is not expected that dietetic intervention would last that long however. Formulate goals of treatment with your patient. This may be only education if the patient is in a contemplative stage of change. It is prudent to set an upper limit to the total number of sessions you will offer (e.g. 12–24 sessions). Reassess the goals and progress on a six-session basis. This will prevent stagnation and allow the dietitian to revise nutrition intervention and consider whether other consultation is needed.

16.3 Patient boundaries

- Expectations of the dietitian's role need to be defined at the start of the intervention. It is useful to discuss the therapeutic limitations of nutrition counseling and to make clear the need for concurrent psychotherapy. Patients need to understand the specific roles of the dietitian dealing with nutrition issues, and those of the professional dealing with psychological issues. Acknowledge that treatment usually entails more than getting a diet plan and that the problem is deeper than the diet. Tell the patient that you believe that there are usually links between food restriction and purging and emotional issues.

- The role of the dietitian is to put back food as nutrition. The overlap between the food restriction or purging and emotions such as suppressed anger or grief may be explored superficially in dietetic sessions but should be the focus of psychological treatment.
- Decide with the patient whether food and emotion diaries are an expectation of treatment. Do not force those who are uncomfortable with keeping records. Recording the food that is ingested and not purged for one or two days may be an acceptable alternative. Patients are encouraged to keep a record of their food intake, purging, activity, and concurrent thoughts, feelings, and emotions.
- State that weight maintenance is a necessary goal at the beginning of treatment. Later, weight gain will be expected. Restoration of a healthy weight is essential to minimize the physical and psychological complications of starvation.
- Make it clear that confidentiality will be kept within the treating team to reduce splitting.
- Admit that you have no magical cure. Promote the importance of the patient assuming an increasing responsibility for recovery.
- State the number of sessions that will be offered before review.

16.4 Dietary history, nutritional assessment, and education

The assessment should include life history, food history, weight history, and an understanding of the patient's view of their problem and how dietetic intervention might help (Table 16.1). An understanding of the role of the illness in the patient's life helps to develop rapport.

Abnormal eating patterns in AN need to be assessed and treated. Nutrition education sessions will help the patient to correct dysfunctional eating patterns, by providing accurate information on a balanced diet, metabolic rate, weight control, how much to eat to gain weight, physical and psychological effects of starvation, food hierarchies of the patient, mood and food, food fears, normal and abnormal eating, activity and weight control, and purging and binge eating.

The stage of motivation to change will affect how weight and food goals are managed. If the patient is just contemplating change, then the initial goals may be limited to weight maintenance and improving food variety.

Table 16.1. *Dietary history and nutritional assessment*

Attitude: client's aims for treatment and motivation to change
Nutrition history Eating patterns and weight history from childhood onwards
Influences on eating and previous nutrition education
Clinical data
Anthropometric data
Biochemical data
Medication and supplements
Social data
Activity pattern
Relevant epidemiology

Example: patient A

When asked whether she had a problem with food and what she expected from seeing the dietitian, the patient's response was as follows:

> Occasionally she thinks she has a problem with her eating disorder. She thinks the issue may be related to anger. She copes with feelings of failure and worthlessness with purging. Vomiting is satisfying, as it helps as an emotional release. Binge eating and vomiting are a means of punishing herself for being "bad." This is more important than the amount of time consumed by the illness.

Patient A is not sure that she wants to be helped into recovery. She cannot see herself without her eating disorder. It is the way she has coped with life. Her psychiatrist wants her to see a dietitian. Sometimes the patient wants help, but she does not want to gain weight.

The session is dominated by the hostility of the patient.

Food, weight, and life history

The patient has had a life of abuse. Her parents suffered from depression and drug abuse. She was told repeatedly that she was either too thin or too fat, but never an acceptable weight. As a child, she was not provided with meals. Eating for comfort sometimes occurred after abusive events in childhood.

The onset of menses and the development of breasts were perceived by the patient as a sign of obesity. Patient A started to binge and vomit during times of anxiety at home.

Her eating disorder is the only stable part of her life and has helped her to cope with her emotions.

Why does the dietitian need to know the personal history?

The patient is in a contemplative stage of change. She is coping with emotions by bingeing and vomiting. The bingeing and vomiting allow her to restrict intake. The dietitian needs to be able to distinguish between a binge that is emotionally or biologically based.

The psychological cause of binge eating and vomiting needs to be acknowledged as part of treatment. The dietitian should not ask for details of abuse. Clearly, this patient should be receiving psychological treatment.

Example: patient B

When asked how she would describe her problem with food and what she wanted from the dietitian, the patient's response was as follows:

> The patient really wanted to get better and was really motivated to change dietary patterns.

Food, weight, and life history

The patient was a young woman of Asian Muslim parents born in the UK. There were a number of difficulties because she was a female and it was the family's first generation in a Western culture. For example, the clothing that was permissible for her to wear was out of keeping with the norm. She began purging and restricting when she was told she could not date her Western boyfriend. She was subsequently sent back to Asia as an act of "cleansing."

Patient B only vomited if she was alone at home. Although she said she wanted to learn to eat normally, dietary change was unlikely to occur without psychological therapy.

Why does the dietitian need to know the personal history?

The patient hoped that the dietitian would rescue her from her eating disorder. The patient was receiving no psychological treatment. Dietetic intervention was one part of treatment, but a team approach, including psychological and family therapy, were needed.

16.5 Specific problems for the dietitian working with eating disordered patients

Professional dilemmas

Dilemmas may arise when treating elite athletes, dancers, and professional singers. Some professions demand a low BMI that would be unhealthy and might precipitate or worsen an eating disorder.

Witnessing distress

It is possible that the dietitian may be the first person to hear stories of abuse or suicidality. Compassion and humanity are qualities that the dietitian needs to help patients with eating disorders. As professionals, dietitians need to acknowledge that witnessing distress is part of the job. Occasionally, however, emotions will surface in their interactions.

Coercion

A patient being treated under the Mental Health Act or guardianship should still be treated with respect and dignity. Maintain non-blaming and non-judgmental interactions. One approach to help explain why tube feeding must be used, against the patient's will, might be to say: "This is required for health reasons. If you had a heart attack, you would not question the doctor's medication. I need to be professional and look after your best health at this moment in time as a requirement of the law. If I don't proceed as to the best of my dietetic abilities, I could be facing negligent charges in court." Explain expectations of weight gain. Do not get involved in debating rates of feed or compromising your clinical judgment in a life-threatening situation.

Families

It takes years of training to become a family therapist. However, dietitians continue to be expected to see families on their own. When possible, try to limit intervention with parents to the beginning and the end of the session.

Clinical supervision

Pedder wrote: "It is a counsel of perfection that no therapist, however experienced, should work without supervision." Clinical supervision has a number of definitions. One definition is: "the encouragement of professional development and growth of clinical practice through the formalized process of meetings between two or more health professionals in which clinical work is discussed."

The dietitian who is not specialized can benefit from dietetic peer review. The specialized dietitian can benefit from a clinical supervisor who works in psychiatry or psychology.

Supervision is needed to maintain and enhance skills, prevent burnout, and document clinical standards. Clinical supervision may also provide a forum for the dietitian to debrief and solve difficulties.

Limitations of a dietitian's involvement

The American Dietetic Association (ADA) position paper of 1994 recommends that treatment by unspecialized dietitians should be time-limited, brief, and focused on nutrition education. The role of the specialist dietitian is also defined by this paper as having contact with the treating multidisciplinary professionals, to regularly communicate with the multidisciplinary team, to have access to clinical supervision, and to have received training in basic counseling skills.

However, in communities where specialist treatment is restricted to the larger cities, it is not always possible to have access to a specialist dietitian.

16.6 Conclusion

The dietician who works with eating disordered patients can fulfill an educational and treatment role. Dietary intervention in these patients will increase emotional distress and will not be effective without psychological treatment. A team approach to treatment is vital. The dietitian should not work alone. To work successfully with eating disorder patients, the dietitian should have clinical supervision (preferably with a psychiatrist or psychologist).

Chapter 17

Information for family and friends

AN is a disease, like asthma is a disease. It is not dieting, a strong wish to be thin, or malingering. People afflicted with AN have within their minds two realities. One reality is a normal and healthy one. Just like you and I, those who suffer from AN want to be happy, healthy, and normal. The other reality is best understood as a phobia, a state of immense fear and concern. In AN, the phobia is that of loss of control, leading to obesity. Just like a phobia of going outside, AN has far-reaching implications. The phobia of personal obesity leads to changes in exercise, eating, unusual behaviors, and an almost constant state of fear, anxiety, and inability to cope with life. The weight loss that results from this phobic state can be life-threatening.

17.1 What causes anorexia nervosa?

Anorexia is a disease that occurs in about one in 100–200 women and about two in 1000 men. The onset of AN is preceded by weight loss. The weight loss may have occurred for any reason, e.g. dieting, travel, diarrhea, or after surgery. AN also requires a certain genetic make-up. AN cannot occur in those who do not have a genetic predisposition to the disease. Even with a genetic predisposition and weight loss, other factors, such as social, environmental, family, or psychological stressors, may be necessary for the disease to manifest itself.

It is best to think of AN as a disease like asthma. Asthma is a genetic disease. It often first manifests itself in the teenage years, like AN. Like AN, asthma is usually precipitated by specific factors. In asthma, these factors may be viral infections or physical causes, such as mold or dust. Asthma is not anyone's fault, and neither is AN.

257

17.2 The course of anorexia nervosa

AN is a disease like asthma, depression, or diabetes. All of these diseases are serious diseases that affect people's lives. They require attention, but they can be treated successfully so that life can be lived happily and productively. All of these diseases may be present for a long time, or even permanently. It takes the average patient with AN seven years to recover. During the course of AN, there are likely to be periods of improvement and periods of worsening, just like in asthma, diabetes, and depression.

17.3 Complications of anorexia nervosa

- Dry skin, rash, hair loss, lanugo hair (fine body hair), hypercarotenemia (yellow skin), Russell's sign (scarring on the back of the hand), blue extremities
- Loss of night vision, difficulty in maintaining visual focus
- Loss of taste or smell, sores at side of mouth, bleeding gums, soreness or erosion of teeth
- Palpitations, chest pains, dizziness, mitral valve prolapse
- Abdominal pain, difficult or painful swallowing, abdominal pain or tenderness
- Confusion or forgetfulness, weakness, seizures, loss of consciousness, muscle spasms, decreased sensations
- Osteoporosis, bone pain, easy fracturing

In people with chronic AN, there will be progressive loss of tissue, including muscle, from the body; memory and concentration will be impaired; vision at night and visual focus may be lessened; the skin will become dry; the heart will become thin and predisposed to palpitations; the bowel will be weakened, resulting in abdominal pains and constipation; the kidneys will not concentrate urine as well as normal, resulting in more frequent urination at night; the bones will become progressively thinner, resulting in bone pain and fractures; and eventually collapse, seizures, and loss of consciousness can occur.

17.4 Recovery

With recovery, the only remaining complications are usually tooth erosion and osteoporosis. If AN starts before the end of adolescence and continues past the time when the growth plates of the bones have closed, then the patient will never reach their maximum potential height. Osteoporosis can continue to get better at any time in life.

17.5 Treatment

AN results in medical problems as well as psychological problems. Treatment must address both medical and psychological problems if it is to be successful. A psychiatrist or psychologist who specializes in AN can provide psychological and family treatment; medical problems including malnutrition must be assessed by a medical doctor and require a dietitian's advice.

Involvement of the patient's family and the use of medications is routine. This does not mean that the family is the cause of the AN or that the medication will be needed forever.

AN is best treated by an eating disorder clinic that consists of a specially trained team of health care workers. Eating assistance and advice, follow-up of physical health concerns, and a variety of specialized psychological treatments may be needed at various stages of treatment. Admission to hospital, medications, formula diets, group therapy, family therapy, and physical therapy may all be required.

17.6 Where can I get information about treatment for anorexia nervosa?

- Start by asking your family doctor.
- Contact the eating disorder resource center in your area, if there is one.
- Contact a university psychiatry department.
- Ask the local medical or psychological association.
- The Internet is a good source of information.

Bibliography

Definitions and epidemiology

Ben-Tovim, D. I., Walker, K., Gilchrist, P., Freeman, R., Kalucy, R. and Esterman, A. Outcome in patients with eating disorders: a 5-year study. *Lancet* 2001; **357**: 1254–7.

Beumont, P. The mental health of young people in Australia: report by the National Mental Health Strategy. *Aust. N. Z. J. Psychiatry* 2002; **36**: 141.

Bryant-Waugh, R., Knibbs, J., Fosson, A., Kaminski, Z. and Lask, B. Long term follow up of patients with early onset anorexia nervosa. *Arch. Dis. Child.* 1988; **63**: 5–9.

Crisp, A. H., Callender, J. S., Halek, C. and Hsu, L. K. Long-term mortality in anorexia nervosa. A 20-year follow-up of the St George's and Aberdeen cohorts. *Br. J. Psychiatry* 1992; **161**: 104–7.

Fairburn, C. G. and Beglin, S. J. Studies of the epidemiology of bulimia nervosa. *Am. J. Psychiatry* 1990; **147**: 401–8.

Fairburn, C. G. and Harrison, P. J. Eating disorders. *Lancet* 2003; **361**: 407–16.

Fichter, M. M. and Quadflieg, N. Six-year course of bulimia nervosa. *Int. J. Eat. Disord.* 1997; **22**: 361–84.

Gull, W. Anorexia nervosa (apepsia hysterica). *Br. Med. J.* 1873; **2**: 527–8.

Hay, P. J., Gilchrist, P. N., Ben-Tovim, D. I., Kalucy, R. S. and Walker, M. K. Eating disorders revisited. II: Bulimia nervosa and related syndromes. *Med. J. Aust.* 1998; **169**: 488–91.

Herzog, W., Deter, H. C., Fiehn, W. and Petzold, E. Medical findings and predictors of long-term physical outcome in anorexia nervosa: a prospective, 12-year follow-up study. *Psychol. Med.* 1997; **27**: 269–79.

Kotler, L. A., Cohen, P., Davies, M., Pine, D. S. and Walsh, B. T. Longitudinal relationships between childhood, adolescent, and adult eating disorders. *J. Am. Acad. Child. Adolesc. Psychiatry* 2001; **40**: 1434–40.

Lasegue, C. De l'anorexie hysterique. *Arch. Gen. Med.* 1873; **2**: 367.

Morande, G., Celada, J. and Casas, J. J. Prevalence of eating disorders in a Spanish school-age population. *J. Adolesc. Health* 1999; **24**: 212–19.

Nilsson, E. W., Gillberg, C., Gillberg, I. C. and Rastam, M. Ten-year follow-up of adolescent-onset anorexia nervosa: personality disorders. *J. Am. Acad. Child. Adolesc. Psychiatry* 1999; **38**: 1389–95.

Steinhausen, H. C. The outcome of anorexia nervosa in the 20th century. *Am. J. Psychiatry* 2002; **159**: 1284–93.

Strober, M., Freeman, R. and Morrell, W. The long-term course of severe anorexia nervosa in adolescents: survival analysis of recovery, relapse, and outcome predictors over 10–15 years in a prospective study. *Int. J. Eat. Disord.* 1997; **22**: 339–60.

Sullivan, P. F., Bulik, C. M. and Kendler, K. S. Genetic epidemiology of binging and vomiting. *Br. J. Psychiatry* 1998; **173**: 75–9.

Theander, S. Outcome and prognosis in anorexia nervosa and bulimia: some results of previous investigations, compared with those of a Swedish long-term study. *J. Psychiatr. Res.* 1985; **19**: 493–508.

Prevention

Buddeberg-Fischer, B., Klaghofer, R., Gnam, G. and Buddeberg, C. Prevention of disturbed eating behaviour: a prospective intervention study in 14- to 19-year old Swiss students. *Acta. Psychiatr. Scand.* 1998; **98**: 146–55.

O'Dea, J. School-based interventions to prevent eating problems: first do no harm. *Eat. Disord. J. Treat. Prev.* 2000; **8**: 123–30.

O'Dea, J. and Abraham, S. Improving body image, eating attitudes, and behaviours of young male and female adolescents: a new educational approach that focuses on self esteem. *Int. J. Eat. Disord.* 2000; **28**: 43–57.

Risk factors

Fairburn, C. G. and Harrison, P. J. Risk factors for anorexia nervosa. *Lancet* 2003; **361**: 1914.

Fairburn, C. G., Cooper, Z., Doll, H. A. and Welch, S. L. Risk factors for anorexia nervosa: three integrated case-control comparisons. *Arch. Gen. Psychiatry* 1999; **56**: 468–76.

Fairburn, C. G., Doll, H. A., Welch, S. L., Hay, P. J., Davies, B. A. and O'Connor, M. E. Risk factors for binge eating disorder: a community-based, case-control study. *Arch. Gen. Psychiatry* 1998; **55**: 425–32.

Fairburn, C. G., Welch, S. L., Doll, H. A., Davies, B. A. and O'Connor, M. E. Risk factors for bulimia nervosa. A community-based case-control study. *Arch. Gen. Psychiatry* 1997; **54**: 509–17.

Frisch, A., Laufer, N., Danziger, Y., *et al.* Association of anorexia nervosa with the high activity allele of the COMT gene: a family-based study in Israeli patients. *Mol. Psychiatry* 2001; **6**: 243–5.

Odent, M. Risk factors for anorexia nervosa. *Lancet* 2003; **361**: 1913–14.

Diagnosis (DSM-IV)

World Health Organization. *Classification of Mental and Behavioural Disorders (ICD-10)*. Geneva: World Health Organization, 1992.

American Psychiatric Association. *Diagnostic and Statistical Manual of Mental Disorders*, 4th edn. Washington, DC: American Psychiatric Association, 1994.

Clinical presentation

Beumont, P. Clinical presentation of anorexia nervosa and bulimia nervosa. In: K. Brownell and C. Fairburn (eds). *Eating Disorders and Obesity*, 2nd edn. New York: Guildford Press, 2002, pp. 162–70.

Beumont, P., George, G. C. W. and Smart, D. E. "Dieters" and "vomiters and purgers" in anorexia nervosa. *Psychol. Med.* 1976; **6**: 617–22.

Beumont, P., Kopec-Schrader, E. and Touyz, S. W. Defining subgroups of dieting disorder patients by means of the Eating Disorders Examination (EDE). *Br. J. Psychiatry* 1995; **166**: 472–4.

Bourne, S. K., Bryant, R. A., Griffiths, R. A., Touyz, S. W. and Beumont, P. J. Bulimia nervosa, restrained, and unrestrained eaters: a comparison of non-binge eating behavior. *Int. J. Eat. Disord.* 1998; **24**: 185–92.

Fairburn, C. G., Cooper, Z., Doll, H. A., Norman, P. and O'Connor, M. The natural course of bulimia nervosa and binge eating disorder in young women. *Arch. Gen. Psychiatry* 2000; **57**: 659–65.

Fisher, M., Schneider, M., Burns, J., Symons, H. and Mandel, F. S. Differences between adolescents and young adults at presentation to an eating disorders program. *J. Adolesc. Health* 2001; **28**: 222–7.

Fosson, A., Knibbs, J., Bryant-Waugh, R. and Lask, B. Early onset anorexia nervosa. *Arch. Dis. Child.* 1987; **62**: 114–18.

Marino, M. F. and Zanarini, M. C. Relationship between EDNOS and its subtypes and borderline personality disorder. *Int. J. Eat. Disord.* 2001; **29**: 349–53.

Pike, K. M. Long-term course of anorexia nervosa: response, relapse, remission, and recovery. *Clin. Psychol. Rev.* 1998; **18**: 447–75.

Rieger, E., Touyz, S. W. and Beumont, P. J. The Anorexia Nervosa Stages of Change Questionnaire (ANSOCQ): information regarding its psychometric properties. *Int. J. Eat. Disord.* 2002; **32**: 24–38.

Course and outcome

Ben-Tovim, D. I., Walker, K., Gilchrist, P., Kalucy, R. and Esterman, A. Outcome in patients with eating disorders: a 5-year study. *Lancet* 2001; **357**: 1254–7.

Fairburn, C. G., Cooper, Z., Doll, H. A., Norman, P. and O'Connor, M. The natural course of bulimia nervosa and binge eating disorder in young women. *Arch. Gen. Psychiatry* 2000; **57**: 659–65.

Russell, G. F. M. The prognosis of eating disorders: a clinician's approach. In: W. Herzog, H. -C. Deter and W. Vandereycken (eds). *The Course of Eating Disorders*. Berlin: Springer-Verlag, 1992, pp. 198–213.

Steinhausen, H. -C. The outcome of anorexia nervosa in the twentieth century. *Am. J. Psychiatry* 2002; **159**: 1284–93.

Theander, S. Chronicity in anorexia nervosa. In: W. Herzog, H. -C. Deter and

W. Vandereycken (eds). *The Course of Eating Disorders*. Berlin: Springer-Verlag, 1992, pp. 214–27.

Physical examination

Birmingham, C. L., Muller, J. L. and Goldner, E. M. Randomized trial of measures of body fat versus body weight in the treatment of anorexia nervosa. *Eat. Weight Disord.* 1998; **3**: 84–9.

Tyler, I. and Birmingham, C. L. The interrater reliability of physical signs in patients with eating disorders. *Int. J. Eat. Disord.* 2001; **30**: 343–5.

Weight and body mass index measurement

Birmingham, C. L., Jones, P. J., Orphanidou, C., *et al.* The reliability of bioelectrical impedance analysis for measuring changes in the body composition of patients with anorexia nervosa. *Int. J. Eat. Disord.* 1996; **19**: 311–15.

Birmingham, C. L., Muller, J. L. and Goldner, E. M. Randomized trial of measures of body fat versus body weight in the treatment of anorexia nervosa. *Eat. Weight Disord.* 1998; **3**: 84–9.

Chen, M. M., Lear, S. A., Gao, M., Frohlich, J. J. and Birmingham, C. L. Intraobserver and interobserver reliability of waist circumference and the waist-to-hip ratio. *Obes. Res.* 2001; **9**: 651.

McCargar, L., Taunton, J., Birmingham, C. L., Pare, S. and Simmons, D. Metabolic and anthropometric changes in female weight cyclers and controls over a 1-year period. *J. Am. Diet. Assoc.* 1993; **93**: 1025–30.

Orphanidou, C. I., McCargar, L. J., Birmingham, C. L. and Belzberg, A. S. Changes in body composition and fat distribution after short-term weight gain in patients with anorexia nervosa. *Am. J. Clin. Nutr.* 1997; **65**: 1034–41.

Orphanidou, C., McCargar, L., Birmingham, C. L., Mathieson, J. and Goldner, E. Accuracy of subcutaneous fat measurement: comparison of skinfold calipers, ultrasound, and computed tomography. *J. Am. Diet. Assoc.* 1994; **94**: 855–8.

Touyz, S. W., Lennerts, W., Freeman, R. J. and Beumont, P. J. To weigh or not to weigh? Frequency of weighing and rate of weight gain in patients with anorexia nervosa. *Br. J. Psychiatry* 1990; **157**: 752–4.

Laboratory testing

Beumont, P. J. and Large, M. Hypophosphataemia, delirium and cardiac arrhythmia in anorexia nervosa. *Med. J. Aust.* 1991; **155**: 519–22.

Cariem, A. K., Lemmer, E. R., Adams, M. G., Winter, T. A. and O'Keefe, S. J. Severe hypophosphataemia in anorexia nervosa. *Postgrad. Med. J.* 1994; **70**: 825–7.

Crow, S. J., Rosenberg, M. E., Mitchell, J. E. and Thuras, P. Urine electrolytes as markers of bulimia nervosa. *Int. J. Eat. Disord.* 2001; **30**: 279–87.

Crow, S. J., Salisbury, J. J., Crosby, R. D. and Mitchell, J. E. Serum electrolytes as markers of vomiting in bulimia nervosa. *Int. J. Eat. Disord.* 1997; **21**: 95–8.

Gambling, D. R., Birmingham, C. L. and Jenkins, L. C. Magnesium and the anaesthetist. *Can. J. Anesth.* 1998; **35**: 644–54.

Hadigan, C. M., Anderson, E. J., Miller, K. K., *et al.* Assessment of macronutrient and micronutrient intake in women with anorexia nervosa. *Int. J. Eat. Disord.* 2000; **28**: 284–92.

Haglin, L. Hypophosphataemia in anorexia nervosa. *Postgrad. Med. J.* 2001; **77**: 305–11.

Hall, R. C., Beresford, T. P. and Hall, A. K. Hypomagnesemia in eating disorder patients: clinical signs and symptoms. *Psychiatr. Med.* 1989; **7**: 193–203.

Kaysar, N., Kronenberg, J., Polliack, M. and Gaoni, B. Severe hypophosphataemia during binge eating in anorexia nervosa. *Arch. Dis. Child.* 1991; **66**: 138–9.

Mira, M., Stewart, P. M., Vizzard, J. and Abraham, S. Biochemical abnormalities in anorexia nervosa and bulimia. *Ann. Clin. Biochem.* 1987; **24**: 29–35.

Pieper-Bigelow, C., Strocchi, A. and Levitt, M. D. Where does serum amylase come from and where does it go? *Gastroenterol. Clin. North. Am.* 1990; **19**: 793–810.

Powers, P. S., Tyson, I. B., Stevens, B. A. and Heal, A.V. Total body potassium and serum potassium among eating disorder patients. *Int. J. Eat. Disord.* 1995; **18**: 269–76.

Stotzer, P. O., Bjornsson, E. S. and Abrahamsson, H. Interdigestive and postprandial motility in small-intestinal bacterial overgrowth. *Scand. J. Gastroenterol.* 1996; **31**: 875–80.

Differential diagnosis

Adams, R., Hinkebein, M. K., McQuillen, M., Sutherland, S., El Asyouty, S. and Lippmann, S. Prompt differentiation of Addison's disease from anorexia nervosa during weight loss and vomiting. *South. Med. J.* 1998; **91**:208–11.

Nussbaum, M. P., Shenker, I. R., Shaw, H. and Frank, S. Differential diagnosis and pathogenesis of anorexia nervosa. *Pediatrician* 1983–85; **12**:110–17.

Medical manifestations by system
Neurological

Amann, B., Schafer, M., Sterr, A., Arnold, S. and Grunze, H. Central pontine myelinolysis in a patient with anorexia nervosa. *Int. J. Eat. Disord.* 2001; **30**: 462–6.

Brewerton, T. D. and George, M. S. Is migraine related to the eating disorders? *Int. J. Eat. Disord.* 1993; **14**: 75–9.

Butow, P., Beumont, P. and Touyz, S. Cognitive processes in dieting disorders. *Int. J. Eat. Disord.* 1993; **14**: 319–29.

Lutte, I., Rhys, C., Hubert, C., *et al.* Peroneal nerve palsy in anorexia nervosa. *Acta Neurol. Belg.* 1997; **97**: 251–4.

Parkin, A. J., Dunn, J. C., Lee, C., O'Hara, P. F. and Nussbaum, L. Neuropsychological sequelae of Wernicke's encephalopathy in a 20-year-old woman: selective impairment of a frontal memory system. *Brain Cogn.* 1993; **21**: 1–19.

Patchell, R. A., Fellows, H. A. and Humphries, L. L. Neurologic complications of anorexia nervosa. *Acta Neurol. Scand.* 1994; **89**: 111–16.

Rechlin, T., Loew, T. H. and Joraschky, P. Pseudoseizure "status". *J. Psychosom. Res.* 1997; **42**: 495–8.

Silber, T. J. Seizures, water intoxication in anorexia nervosa. *Psychosomatics* 1984; **25**: 705–6.

Trummer, M., Eustacchio, S., Unger, F., Tillich, M. and Flaschka, G. Right hemispheric frontal lesions as a cause for anorexia nervosa: report of three cases. *Acta Neurochir. (Wien)* 2002; **144**: 797–801.

Dental

Faine, M. P. Recognition and management of eating disorders in the dental office. *Dent. Clin. North Am.* 2003; **47**:395–410.

George, G. C., Zabow, T. and Beumont, P. J. Letter: scurvy in anorexia nervosa. *S. Afr. Med. J.* 1975; **49**: 1420.

Liew, V. P., Frisken, K. W., Touyz, S. W., Beumont, P. J. and Williams, H. Clinical and microbiological investigations of anorexia nervosa. *Aust. Dent. J.* 1991; **36**: 435–41.

Moynihan, P. and Bradbury, J. Compromised dental function and nutrition. *Nutrition* 2001; **17**: 177–8.

Touyz, S. W., Liew, V. P., Tseng, P., Frisken, K., Williams, H. and Beumont, P. J. Oral and dental complications in dieting disorders. *Int. J. Eat. Disord.* 1993; **14**: 341–7.

Skin

Birmingham, C. L. Hypercarotenemia. *N. Engl. J. Med.* 2002; **347**: 222–3.

Glorio, R., Allevato, M., De Pablo, A., *et al.* Prevalence of cutaneous manifestations in 200 patients with eating disorders. *Int. J. Dermatol.* 2000; **39**: 348–53.

Judd, L. E. and Poskitt, B. L. Pellagra in a patient with an eating disorder. *Br. J. Dermatol.* 1991; **125**: 71–2.

Rushton, D. H. Nutritional factors and hair loss. *Clin. Exp. Dermatol.* 2002; **27**: 396–404.

Schulze, U. M., Pettke-Rank, C. V., Kreienkamp, M., *et al.* Dermatologic findings in anorexia and bulimia nervosa of childhood and adolescence. *Pediatr. Dermatol.* 1999; **16**: 90–94.

Strumia, R., Varotti, E., Manzato, E. and Gualandi, M. Skin signs in anorexia nervosa. *Dermatology* 2001; **203**: 314–17.

Tyler, I., Wiseman, M. C., Crawford, R. I. and Birmingham, L. C. Cutaneous manifestations of eating disorders. *J. Cutan. Med. Surg.* 2002; **6**: 345–53.

Respiratory

Birmingham, C. L. and Tan, A. O. Respiratory muscle weakness and anorexia nervosa. *Int. J. Eat. Disord.* 2003; **33**: 230–33.

Cambell-Taylor, I. Aspiration pneumonia. *N. Engl. J. Med.* 2001; **344**: 1869.

Cook, V. J., Coxson, H. O., Mason, A. G. and Bai, T. R. Bullae, bronchiectasis and nutritional emphysema in severe anorexia nervosa. *Can. Respir. J.* 2001; **8**: 361–5.

Corless, J. A., Delaney, J. C. and Page, R. D. Simultaneous bilateral spontaneous pneumothoraces in a young woman with anorexia nervosa. *Int. J. Eat. Disord.* 2001; **30**: 110–12.

Murciano, D., Rigaud, D., Pingleton, S., Armengaud, M. H., Melchior, J. C. and Aubier, M. Diaphragmatic function in severely malnourished patients with anorexia nervosa. Effects of renutrition. *Am. J. Respir. Crit. Care Med.* 1994; **150**: 1569–74.

Pieters, T., Boland, B., Beguin, C., *et al.* Lung function study and diffusion capacity in anorexia nervosa. *J. Intern. Med.* 2000; **248**: 137–42.

Cardiovascular

Beumont, P. J. and Large, M. Hypophosphataemia, delirium and cardiac arrhythmia in anorexia nervosa. *Med. J. Aust.* 1991; **155**: 519–22.

Casu, M., Patrone, V., Gianelli, M. V., *et al.* Spectral analysis of R-R interval variability by short-term recording in anorexia nervosa. *Eat. Weight Disord.* 2002; **7**: 239–43.

Davidson, A., Anisman, P. C. and Eshaghpour, E. Heart failure secondary to hypomagnesemia in anorexia nervosa. *Pediatr. Cardiol.* 1992; **13**: 241–2.

Franzoni, F., Mataloni, E., Femia, R. and Galetta, F. Effect of oral potassium supplementation on QT dispersion in anorexia nervosa. *Acta Paediatr.* 2002; **91**: 653–6.

Galetta, F., Franzoni, F., Cupisti, A., Belliti, D., Prattichizzo, F. and Rolla, M. QT interval dispersion in young women with anorexia nervosa. *J. Pediatr.* 2002; **140**: 456–60.

Galetta, F., Franzoni, F., Prattichizzo, F., Rolla, M., Santoro, G. and Pentimone, F. Heart rate variability and left ventricular diastolic function in anorexia nervosa. *J. Adolesc. Health* 2003; **32**: 416–21.

Garcia-Rubira, J. C., Hidalgo, R., Gomez-Barrado, J. J., Romero, D. and Cruz Fernandez, J. M. Anorexia nervosa and myocardial infarction. *Int. J. Cardiol.* 1994; **45**: 138–40.

Ho, P. C., Dweik, R. and Cohen, M. C. Rapidly reversible cardiomyopathy associated with chronic ipecac ingestion. *Clin. Cardiol.* 1998; **21**: 780–3.

Isner, J. M., Roberts, W. C., Heymsfield, S. B. and Yager, J. Anorexia nervosa and sudden death. *Ann. Intern. Med.* 1985; **102**: 49–52.

Panagiotopoulos, C., McCrindle, B. W., Hick, K. and Katzman, D. K. Electrocardiographic findings in adolescents with eating disorders. *Pediatrics* 2000; **105**: 1100–105.

Rechlin, T., Weis, M., Ott, C., Bleichner, F. and Joraschky, P. Alterations of autonomic cardiac control in anorexia nervosa. *Biol. Psychiatry* 1998; **43**: 358–63.

Suri, R., Poist, E. S., Hager, W. D. and Gross, J. B. Unrecognized bulimia nervosa: a potential cause of perioperative cardiac dysrhythmias. *Can. J. Anaesth.* 1999; **46**: 1048–52.

Gastrointestinal

Adson, D. E., Mitchell, J. E. and Trenkner, S. W. The superior mesenteric artery syndrome and acute gastric dilatation in eating disorders: a report of two cases and a review of the literature. *Int. J. Eat. Disord.* 1997; **21**: 103–14.

Chiarioni, G., Bassotti, G., Monsignori, A., *et al.* Anorectal dysfunction in constipated women with anorexia nervosa. *Mayo Clin. Proc.* 2000; **75**: 1015–19.

Chun, A. B., Sokol, M. S., Kaye, W. H., Hutson, W. R. and Wald, A. Colonic and anorectal function in constipated patients with anorexia nervosa. *Am. J. Gastroenterol.* 1997; **92**: 1879–83.

De Caprio, C., Pasanisi, F. and Contaldo, F. Gastrointestinal complications in a patient with eating disorders. *Eat. Weight Disord.* 2000; **5**: 228–30.

McClain, C. J., Humphries, L. L., Hill, K. K. and Nickl, N. J. Gastrointestinal and nutritional aspects of eating disorders. *J. Am. Coll. Nutr.* 1993; **12**: 466–74.

Endocrine

Kam, T., Birmingham, C. L. and Goldner, E. M. Polyglandular autoimmune syndrome and anorexia nervosa. *Int. J. Eat. Disord.* 1994; **16**: 101–3.

Levine, R. L. Endocrine aspects of eating disorders in adolescents. *Adolesc. Med.* 2002; **13**: 129–43.

Mantzoros, C. S. Role of leptin in reproduction. *Ann. N. Y. Acad. Sci.* 2000; **900**: 174–83.

Mattingly, D. and Bhanji, S. Hypoglycaemia and anorexia nervosa. *J. R. Soc. Med.* 1995; **88**: 191–5.

Pauly, R. P., Lear, S. A., Hastings, F. C. and Birmingham, C. L. Resting energy expenditure and plasma leptin levels in anorexia nervosa during acute refeeding. *Int. J. Eat. Disord.* 2000; **28**: 231–4.

Stoving, R. K., Hangaard, J. and Hagen, C. Update on endocrine disturbances in anorexia nervosa. *J. Pediatr. Endocrinol. Metab.* 2001; **14**: 459–80.

Wabitsch, M., Ballauff, A., Holl, R., *et al.* Serum leptin, gonadotropin, and testosterone concentrations in male patients with anorexia nervosa during weight gain. *J. Clin. Endocrinol. Metab.* 2001; **86**: 2982–8.

Amenorrhea

Crow, S. J., Thuras, P., Keel, P. K. and Mitchell, J. E. Long-term menstrual and reproductive function in patients with bulimia nervosa. *Am. J. Psychiatry* 2002; **159**:1048–50.

Jamieson, M. A. Hormone replacement in the adolescent with anorexia and hypothalamic amenorrhea – yes or no? *J. Pediatr. Adolesc. Gynecol.* 2001; **14**: 39.

Marcus, M. D., Loucks, T. L. and Berga, S. L. Psychological correlates of functional hypothalamic amenorrhea. *Fertil. Steril.* 2001; **76**: 310–16.

Renal

Alexandridis, G., Liamis, G. and Elisaf, M. Reversible tubular dysfunction that mimicked Fanconi's syndrome in a patient with anorexia nervosa. *Int. J. Eat. Disord.* 2001; **30**: 227–30.

Ishikawa, S., Kato, M., Tokuda, T., *et al.* Licorice-induced hypokalemic myopathy and hypokalemic renal tubular damage in anorexia nervosa. *Int. J. Eat. Disord.* 1999; **26**: 111–14.

Bones and joints

Abella, E., Feliu, E., Granada, I., *et al.* Bone marrow changes in anorexia nervosa are correlated with the amount of weight loss and not with other clinical findings. *Am. J. Clin. Pathol.* 2002; **118**: 582–8.

Audi, L., Vargas, D. M., Gussinye, M., Yeste, D., Marti, G. and Carrascosa, A. Clinical and biochemical determinants of bone metabolism and bone mass in adolescent female patients with anorexia nervosa. *Pediatr. Res.* 2002; **51**: 497–504.

Heer, M., Mika, C., Grzella, I., Drummer, C. and Herpertz-Dahlmann, B. Changes in bone turnover in patients with anorexia nervosa during eleven weeks of inpatient dietary treatment. *Clin. Chem.* 2002; **48**: 754–60.

LaBan, M. M., Wilkins, J. C., Sackeyfio, A. H. and Taylor, R. S. Osteoporotic stress fractures in anorexia nervosa: etiology, diagnosis, and review of four cases. *Arch. Phys. Med. Rehabil.* 1995; **76**: 884–7.

Seibel, M. J. Nutrition and molecular markers of bone remodelling. *Curr. Opin. Clin. Nutr. Metab. Care* 2002; **5**: 525–31.

Soyka, L. A., Misra, M., Frenchman, A., *et al.* Abnormal bone mineral accrual in adolescent girls with anorexia nervosa. *J. Clin. Endocrinol. Metab.* 2002; **87**: 4177–85.

Zipfel, S., Seibel, M. J., Loewe, B., Beumont, P. J., Kasperk, C. and Herzog, W. Osteoporosis in eating disorders: a follow-up study of patients with anorexia nervosa and bulimia nervosa. *J. Clin. Endocrinol. Metab.* 2001; **86**: 5227–33.

Hematological

Kaiser, U. and Barth, N. Haemolytic anaemia in a patient with anorexia nervosa. *Acta Haematol.* 2001; **106**: 133–5.

Lambert, M., Hubert, C., Depresseux, G., *et al.* Hematological changes in anorexia nervosa are correlated with total body fat mass depletion. *Int. J. Eat. Disord.* 1997; **21**: 329–34.

Immune

Corcos, M., Guilbaud, O., Paterniti, S., *et al.* Involvement of cytokines in eating disorders: a critical review of the human literature. *Psychoneuroendocrinology* 2003; **28**: 229–49.

Nova, E., Samartin, S., Gomez, S., Morande, G. and Marcos, A. The adaptive response of the immune system to the particular malnutrition of eating disorders. *Eur. J. Clin. Nutr.* 2002; **56** (suppl 3): S34–7.

Unclassified

Bihun, J. A., McSherry, J. and Marciano, D. Idiopathic edema and eating disorders: evidence for an association. *Int. J. Eat. Disord.* 1993; **14**: 197–201.

Birmingham, C. L., Stigant, C. and Goldner, E. M. Chest pain in anorexia nervosa. *Int. J. Eat. Disord.* 1999; **25**: 219–22.

Genuardi, F. J. and Sturdevant, M. S. Generalized weakness. *Adolesc. Med.* 1996; **7**: 357–9.

Inpatient treatment

Attia, E., Haiman, C., Walsh, B. T. and Flater, S. R. Does fluoxetine augment the inpatient treatment of anorexia nervosa? *Am. J. Psychiatry* 1998; **155**: 548–51.

Beumont, P. J., Kopec-Schrader, E. M. and Lennerts, W. Eating disorder patients at a NSW teaching hospital: a comparison with state-wide data. *Aust. N. Z. J. Psychiatry* 1995; **29**: 96–103.

Griffiths, R., Gross, G., Russell, J., *et al.* Perceptions of bed rest by anorexic patients. *Int. J. Eat. Disord.* 1998; **23**: 443–7.

Touyz, S. W., Beumont, P. J., Glaun, D., Phillips, T. and Cowie, I. A comparison of lenient and strict operant conditioning programmes in refeeding patients with anorexia nervosa. *Br. J. Psychiatry* 1984; **144**: 517–20.

Touyz, S. W., Lennerts, W., Freeman, R. J. and Beumont, P. J. To weigh or not to weigh? Frequency of weighing and rate of weight gain in patients with anorexia nervosa. *Br. J. Psychiatry* 1990; **157**: 752–4.

Day patient treatment

Anzai, N., Lindsey-Dudley, K. and Bidwell, R. J. Inpatient and partial hospital treatment for adolescent eating disorders. *Child. Adolesc. Psychiatr. Clin. North Am.* 2002; **11**: 279–309.

Dalle Grave, R., Ricca, V. and Todesco, T. The stepped-care approach in anorexia nervosa and bulimia nervosa: progress and problems. *Eat. Weight Disord.* 2001; **6**: 81–9.

Rodriguez, C., Fernandez-Corres, B., Perez, M. J., Iruin, A. and Gonzalez-Pinto, A. Partial hospitalization and outcome of anorexia nervosa. *Eur. Psychiatry* 2002; **17**: 236–7.

Thornton, C., Beumont, P. and Touyz, S. The Australian experience of day programs for patients with eating disorders. *Int. J. Eat. Disord.* 2002; **32**: 1–10.

Touyz, S., Thornton, C., Rieger, E., George, L. and Beumont, P. The incorporation of the stage of change model in the day hospital treatment of patients with anorexia nervosa. *Eur. Child. Adolesc. Psychiatry* 2003; **12** (suppl 1): I65–71.

Zipfel, S., Reas, D. L., Thornton, C., *et al.* Day hospitalization programs for eating disorders: a systematic review of the literature. *Int. J. Eat. Disord.* 2002; **31**: 105–17.

Compulsory treatment

Beumont, P. J. Compulsory treatment in anorexia nervosa. *Br. J. Psychiatry* 2000; **176**: 298–9.

Goldner, E., Birmingham, C. and Smye, V. Addressing treatment refusal in anorexia nervosa: clinical, ethical, and legal considerations. In: D. Garner (ed.). *Handbook of Treatment for Eating Disorders.* Los Angeles: Taylor & Francis, 1996, pp. 150–61.

Ramsay, R., Ward, A., Treasure, J. and Russell, G. F. Compulsory treatment in anorexia nervosa. Short-term benefits and long-term mortality. *Br. J. Psychiatry* 1999; **175**: 147–53.

Russell, G. F. Involuntary treatment in anorexia nervosa. *Psychiatr. Clin. North Am.* 2001; **24**: 337–49.

Medical treatment

American Psychiatric Association. Practice guideline for the treatment of patients with eating disorders (revision). *Am. J. Psychiatry* 2000; **157** (suppl): 1–39.

Bakan, R. The role of zinc in anorexia nervosa: etiology and treatment. *Med. Hypotheses* 1979; **5**: 731–6.

Bakan, R., Birmingham, C. L., Aeberhardt, L. and Goldner, E. M. Dietary zinc intake of vegetarian and nonvegetarian patients with anorexia nervosa. *Int. J. Eat. Disord.* 1993; **13**: 229–33.

Beumont, P. J., Arthur, B., Russell, J. D. and Touyz, S. W. Excessive physical activity in dieting disorder patients: proposals for a supervised exercise program. *Int. J. Eat. Disord.* 1994; **15**: 21–36.

Beumont, P. J., Russell, J. D. and Touyz, S. W. Treatment of anorexia nervosa. *Lancet* 1993; **341**: 1635–40.

Birmingham, C. and Goldner, E. Eating disorders. In: Canadian Pharmaceutical Association (ed.). *Therapeutic Choices,* 3rd edn. Ottawa: Canadian Pharmaceutical Association, 2000, pp. 836–42.

Birmingham, C. L., Goldner, E. M. and Bakan, R. Controlled trial of zinc supplementation in anorexia nervosa. *Int. J. Eat. Disord.* 1994; **15**: 251–5.

Davidson, H. and Birmingham, C. The Ulysses agreement. *Eat. Weight Disord.* 2003; **8**: 249–52.

Goldner, E. and Birmingham, C. Treatment of anorexia nervosa. In: D. B. Lumsden and L. Alexander-Mott (ed.). *Understanding Eating Disorders.* Washington, DC: Taylor & Francis, 1994, pp. 135–57.

Gutierrez, E. and Vazquez, R. Heat in the treatment of patients with anorexia nervosa. *Eat. Weight Disord.* 2001; **6**: 49–52.

Gutierrez, E., Vazquez, R. and Boakes, R. A. Activity-based anorexia: ambient temperature has been a neglected factor. *Psychol. Bull. Rev.* 2002; **9**: 239–49.

Kaye, W. H., Nagata, T., Weltzin, T. E., *et al.* Double-blind placebo controlled administration of fluoxetine in restricting- and restricting-purging-type anorexia nervosa. *Biol. Psychiatry* 2001; **49**: 644–52.

Kopala, L. C., Good, K., Goldner, E. M. and Birmingham, C. L. Olfactory identification ability in anorexia nervosa. *J. Psychiatry Neurosci.* 1995; **20**: 283–6.

Kraemer, H. C., Wilson, G. T., Fairburn, C. G. and Agras, W. S. Mediators and moderators of treatment effects in randomized clinical trials. *Arch. Gen. Psychiatry* 2002; **59**: 877–83.

Lear, S. A., Pauly, R. P. and Birmingham, C. L. Body fat, caloric intake, and plasma leptin levels in women with anorexia nervosa. *Int. J. Eat. Disord.* 1999; **26**: 283–8.

Leung, M. and Birmingham, C. L. Food fight: the management of anorexia nervosa and bulimia nervosa. *Pharm. Pract.* 1997; **13**: 62–72.

Russell, J. D., Mira, M., Allen, B. J., *et al.* Protein repletion and treatment in anorexia nervosa. *Am. J. Clin. Nutr.* 1994; **59**: 98–102.

Russell, J. D., Mira, M., Allen, B. J., *et al.* Effect of refeeding and exercise in restoration of body protein in anorexia nervosa. *Basic Life Sci.* 1993; **60**: 207–10.

Su, J. C. and Birmingham, C. L. Zinc supplementation in the treatment of anorexia nervosa. *Eat. Weight Disord.* 2002; **7**: 20–22.

Thien, V., Thomas, A., Markin, D. and Birmingham, C. L. Pilot study of a graded exercise program for the treatment of anorexia nervosa. *Int. J. Eat. Disord.* 2000; **28**: 101–6.

Pharmacological treatment

Colom, F., Vieta, E., Benabarre, A., *et al.* Topiramate abuse in a bipolar patient with an eating disorder. *J. Clin. Psychiatry* 2001; **62**: 475–6.

Glauser, J. Tricyclic antidepressant poisoning. *Cleve. Clin. J. Med.* 2000; **67**: 704–6, 709–13, 717–19.

Mitchell, J. E., Peterson, C. B., Myers, T. and Wonderlich, S. Combining pharmacotherapy and psychotherapy in the treatment of patients with eating disorders. *Psychiatr. Clin. North Am.* 2001; **24**: 315–23.

Zhu, A. J. and Walsh, B. T. Pharmacologic treatment of eating disorders. *Can. J. Psychiatry* 2002; **47**: 227–34.

Refeeding syndrome

Beumont, P. J. V., Russell, J., Touyz, S., *et al.* Intensive nutritional counselling in bulimia nervosa: a role for supplementation with fluoxetine? *Aust. N. Z. J. Psychiatry* 1997; **31**: 514–24.

Birmingham, C. L., Alothman, A. F. and Goldner, E. M. Anorexia nervosa: refeeding and hypophosphatemia. *Int. J. Eat. Disord.* 1996; **20**: 211–13.

Crook, M. A., Hally, V. and Panteli, J. V. The importance of the refeeding syndrome. *Nutrition* 2001; **17**: 632–7.

Fisher, M., Simpser, E. and Schneider, M. Hypophosphatemia secondary to oral refeeding in anorexia nervosa. *Int. J. Eat. Disord.* 2000; **28**: 181–7.

Huang, Y. L., Fang, C. T., Tseng, M. C., Lee, Y. J. and Lee, M. B. Life-threatening refeeding syndrome in a severely malnourished anorexia nervosa patient. *J. Formos. Med. Assoc.* 2001; **100**: 343–6.

Keyes, S., Brozek, J., Henschel, A. and Taylor, H. *The Biology of Human Starvation.* Minneapolis: University of Minnesota Press, 1950.

Kohn, M. R., Golden, N. H. and Shenker, I. R. Cardiac arrest and delirium: presentations of the refeeding syndrome in severely malnourished adolescents with anorexia nervosa. *J. Adolesc. Health* 1998; **22**: 239–43.

Melchior, J. C. From malnutrition to refeeding during anorexia nervosa. *Curr. Opin. Clin. Nutr. Metab. Care* 1998; **1**: 481–5.

Russell, J., Baur, L. A., Beumont, P. J., *et al.* Altered energy metabolism in anorexia nervosa. *Psychoneuroendocrinology* 2001; **26**: 51–63.

Silber, T. Nutrition, immunity, and refeeding. *Am. J. Clin. Nutr.* 1998; **67**: 947–8.

Specific patient populations
Diabetes mellitus

Fairburn, C. G., Peveler, R. C., Davies, B., Mann, J. I. and Mayou, R. A. Eating disorders in young adults with insulin dependent diabetes mellitus: a controlled study. *Br. Med. J.* 1991; **303**: 17–20.

Herpertz, S., Albus, C., Kielmann, R., *et al.* Comorbidity of diabetes mellitus and eating disorders: a follow-up study. *J. Psychosom. Res.* 2001; **51**: 673–8.

Herpertz, S., Albus, C., Lichtblau, K., Kohle, K., Mann, K. and Senf, W. Relationship of weight and eating disorders in type 2 diabetic patients: a multicenter study. *Int. J. Eat. Disord.* 2000; **28**: 68–77.

Nielsen, S., Emborg, C. and Molbak, A. G. Mortality in concurrent type 1 diabetes and anorexia nervosa. *Diabet. Care* 2002; **25**: 309–12.

Rodin, G., Olmsted, M. P., Rydall, A. C., *et al.* Eating disorders in young women with type 1 diabetes mellitus. *J. Psychosom. Res.* 2002; **53**: 943–9.

Geriatrics

Hall, P. and Driscoll, R. Anorexia in the elderly – an annotation. *Int. J. Eat. Disord.* 1993; **14**: 497–9.

Wahlqvist, M. L., Clarke, D. M., Rassias, C. R. and Strauss, B. J. G. Psychological factors in nutritional disorders of the elderly: part of the spectrum of eating disorders. *Int. J. Eat. Disord.* 1999; **25**: 345–8.

Males

Andersen, A. E. and Holman, J. E. Males with eating disorders: challenges for treatment and research. *Psychopharmacol. Bull.* 1997; **33**: 391–7.

Barry, D. T., Grilo, C. M. and Masheb, R. M. Gender differences in patients with binge eating disorder. *Int. J. Eat. Disord.* 2002; **31**: 63–70.

Beumont, P. J., Beardwood, C. J. and Russell, G. F. The occurrence of the syndrome of anorexia nervosa in male subjects. *Psychol. Med.* 1972; **2**: 216–31.

Eliot, A. O. and Baker, C. W. Eating disordered adolescent males. *Adolescence* 2001; **36**: 535–43.

Robb, A. S. and Dadson, M. J. Eating disorders in males. *Child Adolesc. Psychiatr. Clin. North Am.* 2002; **11**: 399–418.

Siegel, J. H., Hardoff, D., Golden, N. H. and Shenker, I. R. Medical complications in male adolescents with anorexia nervosa. *J. Adolesc. Health* 1995; **16**: 448–53.

Touyz, S. W., Kopec-Schrader, E. M. and Beumont, P. J. Anorexia nervosa in males: a report of 12 cases. *Aust. N. Z. J. Psychiatry* 1993; **27**: 512–17.

Overdose

Catterson, M. L., Pryor, T. L., Burke, M. J. and Morgan, C. D. Death due to alcoholic complications in a young woman with a severe eating disorder: a case report. *Int. J. Eat. Disord.* 1997; **21**: 303–5.

Kozyk, J. C., Touyz, S. W. and Beumont, P. J. Is there a relationship between bulimia nervosa and hazardous alcohol use? *Int. J. Eat. Disord.* 1998; **24**: 95–9.

Pregnancy

Abraham, S., Taylor, A. and Conti, J. Postnatal depression, eating, exercise, and vomiting before and during pregnancy. *Int. J. Eat. Disord.* 2001; **29**: 482–7.

Beumont, P. J. Anorexia, LHRH and ovulation. *Med. J. Aust.* 1985; **142**: 77–8.

Beumont, P. and Tam, P. Anorexia nervosa, infertility and pregnancy. *Med. J. Aust.* 2001; **174**: 155–6.

Crow, S. J., Thuras, P., Keel, P. K. and Mitchell, J. E. Long-term menstrual and reproductive function in patients with bulimia nervosa. *Am. J. Psychiatry* 2002; **159**: 1048–50.

Franko, D. L. and Spurrell, E. B. Detection and management of eating disorders during pregnancy. *Obstet. Gynecol.* 2000; **95**: 942–6.

Franko, D. L., Blais, M. A., Becker, A. E., *et al.* Pregnancy complications and neonatal outcomes in women with eating disorders. *Am. J. Psychiatry* 2001; **158**: 1461–6.

Kye, S. L. Pregnancy in women with eating disorders. *Am. J. Psychiatry* 2002; **159**: 1249–50.

Moschos, S., Chan, J. L. and Mantzoros, C. S. Leptin and reproduction: a review. *Fertil. Steril.* 2002; **77**: 433–44.

Norre, J., Vandereycken, W. and Gordts, S. The management of eating disorders in a fertility clinic: clinical guidelines. *J. Psychosom. Obstet. Gynaecol.* 2001; **22**: 77–81.

Children and younger adolescents

Brewerton, T. D. Bulimia in children and adolescents. *Child. Adolesc. Psychiatr. Clin. North Am.* 2002; **11**: 237–56.

Geist, R., Heinmaa, M., Stephens, D., Davis, R. and Katzman, D. K. Comparison of family therapy and family group psychoeducation in adolescents with anorexia nervosa. *Can. J. Psychiatry* 2000; **45**: 173–8.

Kohn, M. and Golden, N. H. Eating disorders in children and adolescents: epidemiology, diagnosis and treatment. *Paediatr. Drugs* 2001; **3**: 91–9.

Patton, G. C., Selzer, R., Coffey, C., Carlin, J. B. and Wolfe, R. Onset of adolescent eating disorders: population based cohort study over 3 years. *Br. Med. J.* 1999; **318**: 765–8.

Pratt, B. M. and Woolfenden, S. R. Interventions for preventing eating disorders in children and adolescents. *Cochrane Database Syst Rev* 2002.

Rudolph, C. D. and Link, D. T. Feeding disorders in infants and children. *Pediatr. Clin. North Am.* 2002; **49**: 97–112.

Areas of special interest

Families

Gowers, S. and North, C. Difficulties in family functioning and adolescent anorexia nervosa. *Br. J. Psychiatry* 1999; **174**: 63–6.

Latzer, Y., Ben-Ari, A. and Galimidi, N. Anorexia nervosa and the family: effects on younger sisters to anorexia nervosa patients. *Int. J. Adolesc. Med. Health* 2002; **14**: 275–81.

Patel, P., Wheatcroft, R., Park, R. J. and Stein, A. The children of mothers with eating disorders. *Clin. Child. Fam. Psychol. Rev.* 2002; **5**: 1–19.

Family doctor

American Academy of Pediatrics. Committee on Adolescence. Identifying and treating eating disorders. *Pediatrics* 2003; **111**: 204–11.

Gurney, V. W. and Halmi, K. A. An eating disorder curriculum for primary care providers. *Int. J. Eat. Disord.* 2001; **30**: 209–12.

Pritts, S. D. and Susman, J. Diagnosis of eating disorders in primary care. *Am. Fam. Physician* 2003; **67**: 297–304.

Riggs, S. Eating disorders in adolescents: role of the primary care physician. *Med. Health R. I.* 1999; **82**: 391–5.

Walsh, J. M., Wheat, M. E. and Freund, K. Detection, evaluation, and treatment of eating disorders: the role of the primary care physician. *J. Gen. Intern. Med.* 2000; **15**: 577–90.

Nursing

Akridge, K. Anorexia nervosa. *J. Obstet. Gynecol. Neonatal Nurs.* 1989; **18**: 25–30.

Bryant, S. O. and Kopeski, L. M. Psychiatric nursing assessment of the eating disorder client. *Top. Clin. Nurs.* 1986; **8**: 57–66.

Wolfe, B. E. and Gimby, L. B. Caring for the hospitalized patient with an eating disorder. *Nurs. Clin. North Am.* 2003; **38**: 75–99.

Dietitian

Blank, S., Zadik, Z., Katz, I., Mahazri, Y., Toker, I. and Barak, I. The emergence and treatment of anorexia and bulimia nervosa. A comprehensive and practical model. *Int. J. Adolesc. Med. Health* 2002; **14**: 257–60.

Psychiatric and psychological treatment

Bachar, E., Latzer, Y., Kreitler, S. and Berry, E. M. Empirical comparison of two psychological therapies. Self psychology and cognitive orientation in the treatment of anorexia and bulimia. *J. Psychother. Pract. Res.* 1999; **8**: 115–28.

Beumont, P. J. V. The behavioural disturbance, psychopathology, and phenomenology of eating disorders. In: H. Hoek, J. Treasure and M. Katzman (eds). *Neurobiology in the Treatment of Eating Disorders.* Chichester, UK: John Wiley & Sons, 1998.

Brambilla, F., Draisci, A. P. A. and Brunetta, M. Combined cognitive-behavioral, psychopharmacological and nutritional therapy in bulimia nervosa. *Neuropsychobiology* 1995; **32**: 68–71.

Dare, C., Eisler, I., Russell, G., Treasure, J. and Dodge, L. Psychological therapies for adults with anorexia nervosa. *Br. J. Psychiatry* 2001; **178**: 216–21.

Eisler, I., Dare, C., Russell, G. F., Szmukler, G., le Grange, D. and Dodge, E. Family and individual therapy in anorexia nervosa. A 5-year follow-up. *Arch. Gen. Psychiatry* 1997; **54**: 1025–30.

Geist, R., Heinmaa, M., Stephens, D., Davis, R. and Katzman, D. K. Comparison of family therapy and family group psychoeducation in adolescents with anorexia nervosa. *Can. J. Psychiatry* 2000; **45**: 173–8.

Gowers, S., Norton, K., Halek, C. and Crisp, A. H. Outcome of outpatient psychotherapy in a random allocation treatment study of anorexia nervosa. *Int. J. Eat. Disord.* 1994; **15**: 165–77.

Kleifield, E. I., Wagner, S. and Halmi, K. A. Cognitive-behavioral treatment of anorexia nervosa. *Psychiatr. Clin. North Am.* 1996; **19**: 715–37.

Le Grange, D. Family therapy for adolescent anorexia nervosa. *J. Clin. Psychol.* 1999; **55**: 727–39.

Mitchell, J. E., Pyle, R. L., Eckert, E. D., Hatsukami, D., Pomeroy, C. and Zimmerman, R. A comparison study of antidepressants and structured intensive group psychotherapy in the treatment of bulimia nervosa. *Arch. Gen. Psychiatry* 1990; **47**: 149–57.

North, C. and Gowers, S. Anorexia nervosa, psychopathology, and outcome. *Int. J. Eat. Disord.* 1999; **26**: 386–91.

Robin, A. L., Siegel, P. T., Moye, A. W., Gilroy, M., Dennis, A. B. and Sikand, A. A controlled comparison of family versus individual therapy for adolescents with anorexia nervosa. *J. Am. Acad. Child. Adolesc. Psychiatry* 1999; **38**: 1482–9.

Touyz, S. and Beumont, P. Behavioural treatment to promote weight gain in anorexia nervosa. In: D. Garner and P. Garfinkel (eds). *Handbook of Treatment for Eating Disorders.* New York: Guilford Press, 1997, pp. 361–71.

Vitousek, K., Watson, S. and Wilson, G. T. Enhancing motivation for change in treatment-resistant eating disorders. *Clin. Psychol. Rev.* 1998; **18**: 391–420.

Phenomenology

Beumont, P. J. V. Clinical presentation of anorexia and bulimia nervosa. In: K. D. Brownell and C. G. Fairburn (eds). *Eating Disorders and Obesity: A Comprehensive Handbook.* 2nd edn. New York: Guilford Press, 2002, pp. 162–70.

Obesity

Birmingham, C. L., Muller, J. L., Palepu, A., Spinelli, J. J. and Anis, A. H. The cost of obesity in Canada. *Can. Med. Assoc. J.* 1999; **160**: 483–8.

Karlsson, J., Persson, L. O., Sjostrom, L. and Sullivan, M. Psychometric properties and factor structure of the Three-Factor Eating Questionnaire (TFEQ) in obese men and women. Results from the Swedish Obese Subjects (SOS) study. *Int. J. Obes. Relat. Metab. Disord.* 2000; **24**: 1715–25.

Lentes, K. U., Tu, N., Chen, H., *et al.* Genomic organization and mutational analysis of the human UCP2 gene, a prime candidate gene for human obesity. *J. Recept. Signal Transduct. Res.* 1999; **19**: 229–44.

Striegel-Moore, R. H. The impact of pediatric obesity treatment on eating behavior and psychologic adjustment. *J. Pediatr.* 2001; **139**: 13–14.

Index

Note: page numbers in *italics* refer to figures and tables. Plates are indicated by Plate number.

277